How to be Good

John Harris is Emeritus Professor of Bioethics at the University of Manchester. His books include: *The Value of Life* (Routledge, 1985), *Wonderwoman and Superman* (OUP, 1992), and *Clones Genes and Immortality* (OUP, 1998). He is the author or editor of twenty books and over three hundred and fifty papers.

How to be Good

The Possibility of Moral Enhancement

John Harris

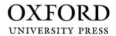
OXFORD
UNIVERSITY PRESS

OXFORD
UNIVERSITY PRESS

Great Clarendon Street, Oxford, OX2 6DP,
United Kingdom

Oxford University Press is a department of the University of Oxford.
It furthers the University's objective of excellence in research, scholarship,
and education by publishing worldwide. Oxford is a registered trade mark of
Oxford University Press in the UK and in certain other countries

© John Harris 2016

The moral rights of the author have been asserted

First published 2016
First published in paperback 2018

Published in the United States of America by Oxford University Press
198 Madison Avenue, New York, NY 10016, United States of America

British Library Cataloguing in Publication Data
Data available

Library of Congress Cataloging in Publication Data
Data available

ISBN 978-0-19-870759-2 (Hbk.)
ISBN 978-0-19-882240-0 (Pbk.)

For Jill Englehart
My wonderful sister who looked after me and looked out for me at a crucial period of my life and remains the best and most generous of friends and mentors.

Contents

Outline of the Book

1. Introduction

This chapter introduces the themes of the book and how they will be developed in succeeding chapters. It explains their importance and their relevance to understanding ethics and to addressing the many moral, political, and policy questions that are being raised by advances in neuroscience, biology, medicine, and robotics. In particular the question "How to be Good?" is introduced and I discuss how the new field of moral enhancement may contribute or fail to contribute to making the world a better place. The question or indeed the task concerning "how to be good" is both an individual and a collective exercise. It involves how an individual can answer such a question with regard to his or her own life and conduct, but also how individual decisions about what to do for the best, which I take to be the paradigmatic moral endeavour, depend on their impact on others and indeed very often on the degree to which others can be prevailed upon to share them and collectively implement them. This joint or collective enterprise is at the heart of social and political action, and of this book.

2. What It's Like to be Good

This chapter discusses how the question: "how to be good?" differs from the question "how to do right?" and considers testing the hypothesis that someone is good, and what thinking about the exercise tells us about goodness and hence of course about how to increase goodness in the world and in people. How in short to answer the question: what is moral enhancement? Here I explore the idea that to act morally is to act for the best "all things considered". In considering what it is like to be good we find that the nature of the good is generic, that what is good for the most part holds good for people across time, culture, and society. This theme pervades the book and is taken up again in the final chapters.

3. Taking the Human out of Human Rights

This chapter takes a step back and looks at the role species membership plays in our conception of rights and also of morality. Is it necessary that moral enhancement applies only to human beings? Might it be legitimate to morally enhance animals or might some very sophisticated machines be persons with rights, responsibilities, and obligations analogous to ourselves? Here we re-examine the concept of human rights, criticize its parochialism, and recommend that if, for convenience, we continue to use the term "human rights" we always bear in mind that we use "human" as a synonym for "person" in John Locke's sense, namely to stand for the sort of creature that "has reason and reflexion and can consider itself the same thinking thing in different times and places".

4. Moral Enhancement and Freedom

God had important things to say on the subject of moral enhancement if God's feelings on the subject have been reliably reported by John Milton. The verbatim account to be found in *Paradise Lost* is important because it contains many of the most cogent reasons for suspicion as to the viability of moral enhancement as a coherent project, not least because of the harm done by existing methods of moral enhancement to the possibility of human freedom as God, Milton, and John Stuart Mill understood that idea. This chapter sets out detailed arguments to show why and how chemical or molecular moral enhancement is essentially inimical to and incompatible with freedom and is therefore unattractive as a device for improving morality or humankind.

5. Taking Liberties with Free Fall

This chapter argues that notions of free will, determinism, and compatibilism are just smoke and mirrors in the context of moral bioenhancement. I make no assumptions about the viability of a non-deterministic account of free will and think some version of compatibilism is probably right. I show here (and indeed throughout this book) that what is at issue is common or garden freedom, the freedom which any rational person accepts is inhibited by threats, diminished by the foreclosure of options, and enhanced by education and civil liberties. I claim that moral bioenhancement acts like a deep-seated irrational prejudice, like racism, sexism, or speciesism. It clouds judgement, making the subject much less able to choose rationally and weigh alternatives from a moral perspective.

6. The God Machine

A crucial issue both in the understanding of the nature of morality and for that reason also in the analysis of what might count as moral enhancement is the role of, indeed the nature of, moral decision-making. Various devices have been from time to time deployed to break the link between thought and action, to show that decisions are not an essential part of the way in which humans connect with the world and hence that responsibility attaches to choices rather than to actions. This chapter examines further one such attempt and notes that while thought and action can be sundered they remain, paradoxically perhaps, inextricably linked in ways that inform our understanding of freedom.

7. "Ethics is for Bad Guys!"

Ethics is for bad guys because the good don't need ethics. The truly good in this sense are so few and far between that few of us ever encounter them. Here it is argued that ethics is principally for those occasions on which compassion, altruism, and basic decency fail; or for those people who fail to do as they should given what will happen to others or to the world if they do not. Moral reasoning is needed to identify the appropriate objects for sympathy, empathy, and the sort of generalized concern, respect, and protection that is the conclusion of a moral argument.

8. Molecules and Morality

Neuroscience is now developing interventions that act directly on the brain influencing behaviour, attitudes, and dispositions, affecting motivation, and, some claim, raising the possibility of adding moral enhancement to physical and cognitive enhancement. These possibilities, if that is what they are, raise important issues of liberty and responsibility which not only affect our sense of who and of what we are, but literally of the extent to which we are, or can remain, masters of our fate, entities which create ourselves by our decisions and actions. This chapter examines and rejects one particularly prominent philosophical argument concerning how to understand the connection between brain function and morality.

9. Moral Progress and Moral Enhancement

This chapter investigates the role of law and regulation on our freedom to act and to affect our conceptions of the good and concludes the dialogue begun in Chapters 6 and 7 with Ingmar Persson and Julian Savulescu about the nature and effects of moral enhancement. One particular point of dispute concerns the relative ease with which harms can be caused as opposed to the alleged difficulty in conferring benefits. I argue that it is self-defeating to use methods, such as those recommended by Persson and Savulescu, that undermine the very capacities required both for moral reflection and judgement but also for moral progress.

10. Mind Reading and Mind Misreading

The idea, the possibility of reading the mind, from the outside, or indeed even from the inside, has exercised humanity from the earliest times. Recent advances in neuroscience have offered some, probably remote, prospect of improved access, but a different branch of technology seems to offer the most promising and the most daunting prospect for both mind reading and mind misreading. You can't have the possibility of the one without the possibility of the other. This chapter tells some of this story. If, and to the extent that we could, read other minds this would be a powerful tool in moral enhancement not least because it might enable the criminal law to anticipate crimes in advance of their commission and resolve vexed problems of intent.

11. The Safety of the People

This chapter sets out in more detail the basis of my optimism about both the varieties of goodness and the many ways in which we can rationally understand how to be good. In discussing a well-established basis for collective or state responsibility for the safety of the people in all its forms, I employ one classic version of what is often called "social contract theory". The social contract is a rational device which further articulates the nature of our mutual moral obligations and responsibilities and places these within a framework which often makes their discharge more manageable, more efficient, and more cost effective. These obligations and responsibilities do not derive from the social contract but rather provide the moral arguments for it, or rather for some instances of it. One conclusion is that the state must act to secure the best for its people, all things considered.

12. Persons or Machines

When considering the further evolution of our species, or for that matter the creation of new species of creatures or of Artificial Intelligence (AI) for existing or future people, it is often assumed that where humans are concerned, those to be enhanced will be and will remain human persons like themselves. Moreover they tend to assume that those people will remain essentially themselves, even in the relevant enhanced state. In short that the modifications in powers and capacities will happen to "us" or those we currently happen to think of as "us". Where we think about the creation of machines or robots with AI we tend to assume that they will remain at our service, literally machines we own and direct, like computers or lawnmowers, and not become persons in their own right. This final chapter considers a possible mechanical rather than organic future for creatures like us.

1

Introduction

We are discussing no trivial subject, but how a man should live

—Plato, *Republic*, 352D[1]

How to be Good? is the pre-eminent question for ethics, although one that philosophers and ethicists seldom address head on. (How this question differs from the question how to do right will be discussed in the next chapter.) Knowing how to be good, or perhaps more modestly and more accurately, knowing how to go about trying to be good, is of immense theoretical and practical importance. It is also perhaps the most important issue facing contemporary neuroscience, social policy, and criminal justice. The links between this highly theoretical question and the preoccupations of contemporary neuroscience and the interests of the criminal law and indeed of those preoccupied with social policy, education, and the common good are all examined in this book. They are examined, however, among other ways, through a lens which focuses on debates about how to effect moral enhancement or moral improvement in human beings.

This lens reveals, I believe, truths (if not the truth) about the nature of morality and of moral action and behaviour, truths which derive from the limitations of the chemical and molecular methods that are believed by many to be effective ways of achieving moral enhancement. We will look at contemporary science, its possibilities and limitations, and examine contemporary debate about the possibilities of using science to alter

---

[1] Quoted by Michael Oakeshott, in his Introduction to: Thomas Hobbes, *Leviathan*, ed. Michael Oakeshott (Oxford: Basil Blackwell, 1960), at p. vii. I guess the translation to be Oakeshott's own and it is one entirely consistent with Plato's philosophy. For a rather different translation of Plato's idea see Benjamin Jowett (ed.), *The Dialogues of Plato* (Oxford: Clarendon Press), volume II, p. 194.

human behaviour for the better and alter human intentions, dispositions, and purposes in analogous ways. This will reveal a picture of what it is to be good which both makes clearer and more accessible what moral improvement, moral education, and indeed what being moral is actually like, and normatively, should actually be like. This investigation will also identify ways to evaluate purported 'scientific' ways of affecting a social and rational institution such as morality.

One, possibly embarrassing, problem with trying to answer the question of how a "man" should live is that:

In the future there will be no more "men" in Plato's sense, no more human beings therefore, and no more planet earth.[2]

Why will there be no more human beings to think about how we should live? Either we will have been wiped out by our own foolishness or by brute forces of nature or, I hope, we will have further evolved by a process more rational and much quicker than Darwinian evolution—a process I described in my book *Enhancing Evolution*.[3] Even more certain it is that there will be no more planet earth. Our sun will die and with it all possibility of life on this planet.

By the time this happens, we may hope that our better evolved successors will have developed the science and the technology needed to survive and to enable us (them) to find and colonize another planet or perhaps even to build another planet; and in the meanwhile to cope better with the problems presented by living on this planet. Most importantly perhaps the problem of how to be good, or how to be good enough to ensure the survival of what may be the only sorts of beings anywhere in the universe capable of caring about their own survival and the survival of others.

If, *In the future there will be no more "men" in Plato's sense, no more human beings therefore, and no more planet earth*, some might ask: what then would be the point of being good and trying to make moral progress? This is an immense question but it has a very obvious and perhaps ultimately unsatisfying if not unsatisfactory answer. Questions

---

[2] Adapted from a remark developed with my friend and colleague John Sulston for a public lecture we gave on 12 May 2008 at The Sheldonian Theatre in Oxford entitled "What is Science For?"

[3] John Harris, *Enhancing Evolution* (Princeton and Oxford: Princeton University Press, 2008).

like this arise really only for people who affect to believe that we have no prudential interest for ourselves, or for the immediate welfare of others. These matters are discussed in more detail in the next chapter. Decisions are both self-changing and self-creating and are also world-changing and world-creating, that is why we make decisions; and if they did not have this effect there would be no point in making them. Decision-making changes us and the world forever. Even if we and the world cease to exist it will have been different because we existed and affected it however briefly and however trivially. But moral decisions are not trivial, they are about making the lives of others and the world a better place, not forever maybe, but not for nothing either. It is tempting to think that individual death and the death of worlds makes all life pointless. I do not believe so: the point lies in the nature of the difference made, for however long that difference lasts and however limited in scope or duration that difference might be. Whether we like it or not we have an effect; the moral question is how we judge the effect of that effect. To this question we return throughout this book.

Stephen Hawking initially predicted that we might have about 7.6 billion years to go before the earth gives up on us; but he recently revised his position in relation to the earth's continuing habitability as opposed to its physical survival:

"We must also continue to go into space for the future of humanity," he said recently. "I don't think we will survive another thousand years without escaping beyond our fragile planet. I therefore want to encourage public interest in space, and I've been getting my training in early."[4]

Martin Rees is famous for (among many other things) his elevation of the "village idiot" to global status. In his fascinating book *Our Final Century*,[5] Rees catalogues the disasters which might, if the causes of them are not addressed, lead to the end of human life on this planet. Rees

---

[4] Stephen Hawking famously estimated we have about 7.6 billion years to go: <http://bigthink.com/dangerous-ideas/5-stephen-hawkings-warning-abandon-earth-or-face-extinction>. Hawking recently revised this estimate with a different event horizon: <http://www.theguardian.com/science/2013/nov/12/stephen-hawking-physics-higgs-boson-particle>. Different recent studies indicate that a realistic figure would be 2.8 billion years: <http://arxiv.org/pdf/1210.5721v1.pdf>.

[5] Martin Rees, *Our Final Century* (London: Arrow Books, 2004).

considers the role of malevolence or wickedness but also warns of the dangers posed by incompetence or stupidity.

We are entering an era when a single person can, by one clandestine act, cause millions of deaths or render a city uninhabitable for years, and when a malfunction in cyberspace can cause havoc worldwide to a significant segment of the economy: air transport, power generation, or the financial system. Indeed disaster could be caused by someone who is merely incompetent rather than malign.[6]

Rees glossed these remarks at the Hay festival in 2006: "in a global village there will be global village idiots, just one could be too many" and he concluded "I think there is a real concern about whether our civilization can be safe-guarded without us having to sacrifice too much in terms of privacy, diversity and individualism."[7] I agree with Rees about this, and would add dangers to liberty and autonomy.

So with all these dangers how can we try to secure the safety of the people, whether these people are human, post human, part human and part animal, part human and part machine or entirely beings with artificial intelligence, mechanical beings who (which) reproduce by mechanical construction, perhaps aided by 3D printers?

1.1 The Safety of the People

The question or indeed the task concerning "how to be good" is both an individual and a collective exercise. It involves how an individual can answer such a question with regard to his or her own life and conduct, but also how individual decisions about what to do for the best, which I take to be the paradigmatic moral endeavour, depend on their impact on others and indeed very often on the degree to which others can be prevailed upon to share them and collectively implement them. This joint or collective enterprise is at the heart of social and political action, to which we return in Chapter 9, but it is worth reminding ourselves at the start that this combination of individual and collective responsibility provides the moral and theoretical basis for both moral and political theory however abstract or philosophical it may become.

---

[6] Rees, *Our Final Century*, p. 61.
[7] As reported in *Guardian Unlimited*, Monday, 29 May 2006.

Sometime before 1651, Thomas Hobbes *of* Malmesbury (but not *in* Malmesbury—probably in Paris where at the time he was tutor to the exiled Charles Prince of Wales)—proposed this wonderful thesis:

> The office of the sovereign, be it a monarch or an assembly, consisteth in the end for which he was trusted with the sovereign power, namely the procuration of *the safety of the people*; to which he is obliged by the law of nature.[8]

This is perhaps the most compelling statement not only of the moral relations between the citizen and the state, and between citizens and one another, but of the foundations of any social contract (real, fictional, or rational) worthy of respect. It is not an accident that Hobbes talks of the safety of the citizenry being *the end for which he* (the ruler) *was trusted with the sovereign power*, by the people who are the source of this power. It may be an elaboration of Marcus Aurelius' famous meditation on his own role as absolute ruler of a vast empire: "A king's lot: to do good and be damned".[9] In short it states the minimum conditions for a legitimate state and in doing so relies on the most basic and fundamental of values, a value which is the prerequisite of what might be thought of as derivative or dependent values, such as happiness, liberty, rights, and justice.

But note that in Hobbes's version of the social contract, to which we return in Chapter 11, the moral obligation to provide for the safety of the people is not a *product of* the social contract, rather it is the *reason for* the social contract. This moral obligation of mutual protection does not arise from the social contract, it is the very reason and justification for establishing the contract in the first place or rather for recognizing that such a contract between people, between moral agents, has always existed. It arises, as we will discuss further in the next chapter and in Chapters 11 and 12, from the nature of the individuals involved. As Ludwig Wittgenstein (perhaps not most renowned for his moral philosophy) remarked:

> My attitude to him is an attitude towards a soul. I am not of the *opinion* that he has a soul.[10]

---

[8] Hobbes, *Leviathan*, p. 145. The details of Hobbes's life I take from Michael Oakeshott's Introduction to this volume, pp. vii ff. We will return to Hobbes in more detail in Chapter 11.

[9] Marcus Aurelius, *Meditations*, trans. Martin Hammond, with an Introduction by Diskin Clay (London: Penguin Books, 2006), Book 7, 36, p. 63.

[10] Ludwig Wittgenstein, *Philosophical Investigations*, trans. G. E. M. Anscombe (Oxford: Basil Blackwell, 1968), Part II, IV, p. 178e.

The value of which we speak is personal and public safety; safety from arbitrary and ill usage by all...from the Sovereign power to the most vicious outlaw, safety also from other sources of terror—from want and disease, hunger and poverty, insofar as these are possible to secure. And safety also from the various apocalyptic threats that in our own time, more than ever before, face every living creature on our planet.

Concern for the safety of the people reflects the value we accord to life itself but also the special value possessed by certain sorts of lives, the lives of persons.[11] It is expressed in our respect for persons, individually and collectively; understood not simply in terms of bare preservation of life, but as a combination of concern for their welfare and respect for their wishes.

Individually it is enshrined in the safety afforded by respect for rights and interests in normative systems as diverse as codes of good manners and politeness, through legal constraints on assault and violation to broad issues of human rights and justice.

It is manifest in health care systems like the British NHS, social welfare provision, and measures of public health and safety from clean water to unemployment benefit and from vaccination and terminal care to product liability and safety at work.

All of these social norms, practices, and institutions are non-explicit and perhaps unconscious measures of the value of life: they are telling us *that* we value it and to an extent *how* and *how much* we value it. But also, and this is why I introduce this idea at the beginning of this book, they tell us about the aims and purposes of morality, of the pre-conditions for a moral life and hence about what moral enhancement might be like and what attempts to achieve moral enhancement must not be like. These issues will reappear and I hope be resolved in Chapter 10.

Understanding the meaning and effect of all this is our project.

The exploration and analysis of the nature and effects of various proposed methods of moral enhancement will reveal important features of the nature of morality and hence ways in which those who wish to enhance their own moral behaviour or who simply want to be good, can rationally try to achieve this.

---

[11] I have given accounts of this peculiar value elsewhere: John Harris, *The Value of Life* (London: Routledge, 1985).

In short, this book will show how we might sensibly try to be good and what methods can or cannot achieve this, for ourselves or others. By doing so we can also show the extent to which 'others', the state, the criminal law, employers, or parents might legitimately attempt to influence behaviour for the better or worse. Finally the book will demonstrate the fallacy of equating so-called "pro-social" or non-aggressive behaviour with moral behaviour, and equally the fallacy of thinking that judgements about issues of moral significance are the same thing as moral judgements. It will be argued that while "being good" is a matter for private morality, "doing good" always addresses public morality in ways that reinforce the account of what it is to be good that this book will deliver.

Human enhancement has become one of the key areas of contemporary science and innovation and a focus of concerns about the responsible and ethical application of science. Until recently both science and innovation and the societal concerns these have occasioned have focused on the enhancement of what might be termed human powers and capacities and on the effect the enhancement of such powers and capacities might have on our understanding of what it is to be human and on the development of society and our world. This has embraced issues such as cognitive enhancement, longevity and immortality, machine–brain interfaces, prosthetics, cosmetic surgery, and "doping"[12] in sport. These have in turn raised questions and concerns about just how far we might deliberately influence the further evolution of humankind to the point where we, or our successors, might cease to be human. I have devoted two previous books to different dimensions of these issues (*Wonderwoman and Superman: The Ethics of Human Biotechnology*, Oxford University Press, 1992, and *Enhancing Evolution*, Princeton University Press, 2007).

Now neuroscience is developing interventions that act directly on the brain, influencing behaviour, attitudes, and dispositions, affecting motivation, and, some claim, raising the possibility of adding moral enhancement to physical and cognitive enhancement. These possibilities, if that is what they are, raise important issues of liberty and responsibility which not only affect our sense of who and of what we are, but literally of the

---

[12] An unnecessarily pejorative term but one that has some currency.

extent to which we are, or can remain, masters of our fate, entities which create ourselves by our decisions and actions.

A recent report of the Royal Society, one of the UK's national academies of science, of which I was a co-author, put it thus:

> The human brain is not viewed in the same way as other organs. The brain holds the key to mind and behaviour, and so to most it has a 'special' status. The relatively young field of neuroscience is the study of the brain and nervous system. The law is concerned with regulating behaviour, and so it is reasonable to ask whether and if so how neuroscience could or should inform the law.[13]

In addition of course to the interest of the law in criminal and moral responsibility and in what the brain might tell us about past, and predictable future, actions, we all have an interest, both for ourselves and others, in the way in which behaviour and dispositions to act might be influenced for better or worse. In short, how moral enhancement and its opposite might be able to affect our present and future behaviour.

In this book I argue, in passing, for the continuation of the enhancement project and for the wisdom of pursuing all forms of enhancement, but the focus is on moral enhancement. In Chapters 1, 2, and 3, I set out my conception of the nature of morality and moral reasoning and the good reasons and arguments there are for thinking that while such a process may for now be principally and characteristically a human activity, this is not necessarily the case, nor can such concerns continue to be confined to our species as presently constituted. In later chapters this conception will be refined by engagement with a number of scholars who argue to the contrary.

Throughout this book I argue that the methods of moral enhancement, considered by these and other contemporary advocates of a specific agenda of moral enhancement, not only may pose dangers to our freedom both of thought and of deed, but will ultimately fail. This failure will be due, I suggest, to a somewhat limited view of the nature of morality, and because the methods of moral enhancement they advocate will be in conflict with, rather than complementary to, the powerful armoury of ways we already have of learning, developing, improving, and deploying our public and private morality. If I am right to suggest

---

[13] The Royal Society, *Brain Waves Module 4: Neuroscience and the Law.* ISBN: 978-0-85403-932-6, December 2011, p. iii. See also *Brain Waves Module 1.* ISBN: 978-0-85403-879-4.

that doing good in the moral sense of that term, involves acting for the best "all things considered" (as argued in the next chapter) then the ability to consider the relevant things will be vital. The ways of improving our cognitive functioning so that we are capable of considering as many of the relevant 'things' as possible are myriad. Such methods include of course education, formal or informal, domestic and institutional, the cultivation and satisfaction of curiosity and scepticism, and also the use of cognition-enhancing drugs, which I have discussed at length in *Enhancing Evolution* and elsewhere. They will also involve, as the subsequent chapters will demonstrate, the refinement and practice of other cognitive tools, such as rationality aided by familiar methods by which the rational consideration of the world is improved: scientific method, philosophy, and other disciplined approaches to the understanding of ourselves and the world. These of course include: medical science, social science, history, literature, art, and the other "human sciences". Other technological enhancements of these familiar "tools", for want of a better term, will of course play their part. These will include the use of technology and Artificial Intelligence in many forms.

Already brain–machine interfaces of various sorts are commonplace. Some of these hardly appear to be anything so sophisticated as constituting an "interface": mobile smartphones, computers, or tablets for example. Even more dramatic examples, or more dramatic uses of familiar examples, are envisaged and indeed are on the way. These will be discussed in the final three chapters.

Contemporary gurus such as Elon Musk and Stephen Hawking have in mind, and have some reservations about, the creation of intelligent machines (Chapter 9). A problem, to be discussed in Chapter 12, arises if we are successful in producing intelligent machines: then such intelligent machines, like sufficiently intelligent animals, would at first sight seem to be persons properly so called and would apparently have whatever rights, responsibilities, and duties are the destiny of all persons including ourselves. They, if and once they exist (Chapter 2 and Chapter 9), might join and help shape the moral community.[14]

Finally some words by way of apology. The way this book has been envisaged and has developed will necessarily involve some small

---

[14] <http://www.nytimes.com/2015/01/11/magazine/death-by-robot.html?_r=3>, accessed 18 January 2015.

elements of repetition for which I thought I should apologize in advance. However, on re-reading the *Meditations* of Marcus Aurelius I came across this bold defence of repetition in the elegant Introduction by Diskin Clay.

The reader will encounter a great deal of repetition in the *Meditations*. This might strike the reader as a stylistic flaw, but for a philosopher seeking to guide himself repetition is a philosophical virtue. Repetition is a form of spiritual exercise designed to reinforce the main principles of Marcus' philosophy; its purpose is to effect a 'dyeing of the soul' (5.16.). Three of the lost common imperatives Marcus addresses to himself are: 'Remember', Keep in mind', 'Do not forget.'[15]

Such thoughts comforted me somewhat until I remembered the lines of Bob Dylan in "Bob Dylan's 115th Dream":[16]

I said, "They refused Jesus, too," he said, "You're not him."

With the awareness of the fact that I am not Marcus Aurelius nor even Diskin Clay, I can only, after due consideration, apologize for such, I hope minimal, repetition that has survived and turn to the fundamental question, asked by Socrates and Plato, presupposed by Marcus Aurelius and now to receive some modest further attention. The question of: How to be good? In asking this question we perhaps should bear in mind the sorts of creatures we are, and the limitations our nature may impose. These limitations will be commented on in the course of this book as they force themselves on our attention. One feature of our evolved nature has been an advantage to us and may help to explain why ethics has always been at the centre of the human agenda. Philip Pullman put it this way:

Cuckoos are irresponsible birds by human standards; they lay their eggs in other birds' nests, and the young cuckoos, when they emerge from the egg, shove their foster brothers and sisters over the edge with no conscience at all, and swallow every worm that the responsible foster mother brings. They don't set us a good example at all. Of course, there isn't a moral dimension here, really: the cuckoo does it because that's the sort of bird she is. And the bird that made the nest

---

[15] Marcus Aurelius, *Meditations*, p. xviii.
[16] <http://www.nstp.de/nstp/texte/dylan/bring_it_home/115.html>, accessed 16 January 2015.

doesn't feed the new chick because she's overflowing with compassion: she can't help what she does. That's the sort of bird she is.

But whether or not it's the business of nature to provide us with moral examples, human beings have been taking moral examples from nature for thousands of years. We can take moral lessons from anything: that's the sort of birds we are.[17]

---

[17] Philip Pullman, "Writing is Despotism, but Reading is Democracy", *New Humanist*, 19 January 2015: <https://newhumanist.org.uk/articles/4799/writing-is-despotism-but-reading-is-democracy>, accessed 4 February 2015.

2

What It's Like to be Good
Individual Responsibility

[I learned from Apollonius] ... moral freedom, the certainty to
ignore the dice of fortune, and have no other perspective, even for
a moment, than that of reason alone ...

Marcus Aurelius, Meditations, Book I, p. 4[1]

When someone says "I'm good thank you!", usually in response to a
polite "How are you?", but often as a way of refusing some request—
"Would you like some more food?", "Can I help you?" and the like—I am
tempted, and often do, respond: "That's an interesting hypothesis—how
are we going to test it?"[2]

A similar thought occurred to Amartya Sen. In his book *The Idea of
Justice* he writes:

I am, of course, aware that modern transatlantic usage has drowned the distinction between 'being good' as a moral quality and 'being well' as a comment on a
person's health (no aches and pains, fine blood pressure, and so on), and I have
long ceased worrying about the manifest immodesty of those of my friends who,
when asked how they are reply with apparent self-praise, 'I am very good.'[3]

This chapter, indeed this book, is about testing that hypothesis: the
hypothesis that someone is good. How might such a claim be tested

---

[1] Marcus Aurelius, *Meditations*, trans. Martin Hammond, with an Introduction by
Diskin Clay (London: Penguin Books, 2006), p. 4.

[2] This chapter draws on John Harris, "What It's Like to be Good", *Cambridge Quarterly
of Healthcare Ethics*, vol. 21, no. 3 (2012): 293–305.

[3] Amartya Sen, *The Idea of Justice* (London: Penguin Books, 2009), p. 31. I am indebted
to John Coggon for reminding me of this.

and sustained and what does thinking about the exercise tell us about goodness and hence of course about how to increase goodness in the world and in people? The answers to these questions will give us important information and insights into what it might be like to attempt to improve our own or our society's morality, what it might be to achieve moral enhancement. Of course neither happiness nor preference satisfaction exhaust the possibilities of good and harm to self and others. Unfairness and injustice as well as assaults on dignity and the entitlement to equal concern, respect, and protection are all varieties of the ways in which good and evil occur.

The questions about how to test the hypothesis that someone is good and how to make it more likely that people will be more consistently good, are perhaps the most important questions facing moral philosophy today. If we can answer them, the answers will not only tell us important things about how to be ethical but also about how to distinguish between the many extravagant claims that are being made about the best strategies for moral improvement both individual and collective. In coming chapters the many highly dubious moral claims that are being made for science-based short cuts to moral improvement and to answers to the question how to create better societies and better people will be examined. First though we must return to our starting hypothesis that someone is a good person or some thing is a good, right thing to do.

Now of course we might try to test the hypothesis by asking the individual making the claim exactly what she had done that was so good and maybe, more sophisticatedly, how she knew she was good or that what she had done or achieved was good and what entitled her to be so sure?

In answer, she might of course claim to be existentially good, good in herself, perhaps because she was full of good intentions, replete with virtues or whatever. Why this is a less plausible, or perhaps a less testable, sort of claim is a point to which we shall return. For the moment let's concentrate on good deeds.

She might instead point to the good she had done or planned to do. The list of good things she might have done and hence might cite in answer to our question would probably be uncontroversial because there is significant consensus about the generic nature of good and bad deeds.

It is genuinely uncontroversial to believe that preventing harm, ameliorating pain or suffering, saving lives, curing the sick or their opposites are good or bad things to do. Equally, treating others unfairly or unjustly or in ways which attack their dignity and standing as equals in the community are equally uncontroversial ways of doing harm. But just as "good reasons must of force give place to better",[4] so likewise with good deeds. Even a good deed done might displace a better that might have been done. So even deeds that might seem "good in themselves" might not be "good all things considered", might not be moral because something better might have been (should have been) considered and done instead.

This is one important reason why strategies for moral enhancement,[5] that is to say, strategies which involve *engineering, programming*, or *compelling* moral improvement,[6] rather than strategies for simply educating, training, or encouraging it, may be missing an important point. These will be examined in detail in later chapters. For the moment it is sufficient to note that these strategies propose operating directly on the alleged mainsprings of action, on emotions or other dispositions. In particular that they operate by cutting out or bypassing what they perceive as a dangerously paralysing or dilatory process which might somehow get between an impulse and the moral action it impels. This sometimes, but not necessarily always, dilatory process is thought or reflection. Indeed thought is

---

[4] William Shakespeare, *Julius Caesar*, Act 4, Scene 3. Brutus is addressing Cassius. The Arden Shakespeare, *Complete Works*, ed. Richard Proudfoot, Ann Thomson, and David Scott Kastan (Walton-on-Thames: Thomas Nelson and Sons, 1998).

[5] Thomas Douglas, "Moral Enhancement", *Journal of Applied Philosophy*, vol. 25, no. 3 (2008): 228–45; Ingmar Persson and Julian Savulescu, "The Perils of Cognitive Enhancement and the Urgent Imperative to Enhance the Moral Character of Humanity", *Journal of Applied Philosophy*, vol. 25, no. 3 (2008): 162–77. See also John Harris, "Moral Enhancement and Freedom", *Bioethics*, vol. 25, no. 2 (2011): 102–11; Molly J. Crockett, Luke Clark, Marc D. Hauser, and Trevor W. Robbins, "Serotonin Selectively Influences Moral Judgment and Behavior through Effects on Harm Aversion", *Proceedings of the National Academy of Sciences USA*, vol. 107, no. 40 (2010): 17433–8; John Harris and Sarah Chan, "Moral Behaviour is Not What It Seems", *Proceedings of the National Academy of Sciences USA*, Early Edition (2010): <http://www.pnas.org/cgi/doi/10.1073/pnas.1015001107>; Sarah Chan and John Harris, "Moral Enhancement and Prosocial Behaviour", *Journal of Medical Ethics*, vol. 37, no. 3 (2011): 130–1.

[6] Julian Savulescu and Ingmar Persson, "Moral Enhancement, Freedom and the God Machine", *The Monist*, vol. 95, no. 3 (2012): 399–421. Available at: <http://www.ncbi.nlm.nih.gov/pmc/articles/PMC3431130/>, accessed 21 January 2014.

proverbially and paradoxically paralysingly slow and dynamically fast—"quick as thought"!

2.1 People Matter

I am talking here of what is good or bad for persons, about welfare; but also about justice and rights and responsibilities, all of which I take to be dimensions of welfare broadly conceived. Right and wrong, in short morality, matter because people matter. Elsewhere I have developed a theory of personhood which attempts to explain what sorts of being persons are and why their existence has value.[7] It is not of course only persons that matter morally, but they matter in a different and more significant way than say, most animals, and in this book I am concerned with what it is for people to be good and what is good for people.

In the opening chapter of his magisterial two-volume book *On What Matters*, Derek Parfit says:[8]

We are the animals that can both understand and respond to reasons. These abilities have given us great knowledge, and power to control the future of life on Earth. Though there may be life elsewhere, there may be no other animals like us. We may be the only rational beings in the Universe . . .

It is hard to explain the *concept* of a reason, or what the phrase 'a reason' means. Facts give us reasons, we might say, when they count in favour of our having some attitude, or our acting in some way. But 'counts in favour of' means roughly 'gives a reason for'. Like some other fundamental concepts, such as those involved in our thoughts about time, consciousness, and possibility, the concept of a reason is indefinable in the sense that it cannot be helpfully explained by using words. We must explain such concepts in a different way, by getting people to think thoughts that use these concepts. One example is the thought that we always have a reason to want to avoid being in agony.

It is significant that Parfit chooses here a state that we all have a reason to want to avoid, a state which is thus objectively bad. Before exploring

---

[7] John Harris, *Violence and Responsibility* (London: Routledge & Kegan Paul, 1980); John Harris, *The Value of Life* (London: Routledge & Kegan Paul, 1985), Chapter 1; and John Harris, "The Concept of the Person and the Value of Life", *Kennedy Institute of Ethics Journal*, vol. 9, no. 4 (1999): 293–308.

[8] Derek Parfit, *On What Matters, Volume One* (Oxford: Oxford University Press, 2011), p. 31.

some others of such states we should note that at the end of this volume Parfit returns to the possibility that creatures like us might be unique in the universe, and to a theme that I addressed in the first chapter of my last book,[9] the uncertainty of the future for creatures like us. He concludes:

> What now matters most is that we rich people give up some of our luxuries, ceasing to overheat the Earth's atmosphere, and taking care of this planet in other ways, so that it continues to support intelligent life. If we are the only rational animals in the Universe, it matters even more whether we shall have descendants in the billions of years in which that would be possible. Some of our descendants might live lives and create worlds that, though failing to justify past suffering, would give us all, including those who suffered, reasons to be glad that the Universe exists.[10]

It is to the nature of those reasons to be glad that we must now turn.

2.2 The Generic Character of the Good

I have suggested that the nature of the good is well understood, is moreover "generic", and that there is considerable consensus as to the nature of the good, considerable consensus as to what we have to be pleased about. This requires some amplification.

It is often fruitful to attempt to define things in terms of their opposites. Some time ago I defined disability as a harmed condition that someone has a strong rational preference not to be in, harmed not relative to what is normal or species typical, but relative to what is known to be possible.[11] I was looking for a definition that would be adaptable to changing ideas of health and disease, and which would make sense of the

---

[9] John Harris, *Enhancing Evolution* (Princeton and Oxford: Princeton University Press, 2007).

[10] Parfit, *On What Matters, Volume 1*, p. 419. On the subject of time, Stephen Hawking famously estimated we have about 7.6 billion years to go: <http://bigthink.com/dangerous-ideas/5-stephen-hawkings-warning-abandon-earth-or-face-extinction>. But more recent studies indicate that a realistic figure would be 2.8 billion years: <http://arxiv.org/pdf/1210.5721v1.pdf>.

[11] Here the discussion follows lines taken in Harris, *Enhancing Evolution*. For more distant roots of this idea see John Harris, "Is Gene Therapy a Form of Eugenics?", *Bioethics*, vol. 7, no. 2–3 (1993): 178–88. See also my discussion of the difference between harming and wronging: John Harris, *Wonderwoman and Superman: The Ethics of Human Biotechnology* (Oxford: Oxford University Press, 1992), Chapter 4.

idea that continuing human enhancement might make us come to think of those who, perhaps say, by the standards of 1984, were not damaged, diseased, injured, or harmed in any way, were none the less hampered, effectively disabled, relative to their enhanced contemporaries. In other words there were powers and capacities that had become available and were perhaps becoming "normalized" (or were in danger of not becoming normalized to the detriment of all), but which they lacked.[12]

The Janus face of this definition is that the opposite of a harmed condition which we have a strong rational preference not to be in, is a healthy or beneficial condition that we have a strong rational preference to be and remain in. That condition, in health terms, is one that is the opposite of being disabled, being in a harmful condition, which is of course being fit and healthy, being in good condition. Conditions which it would be good, morally speaking, to help others to attain and maintain and would also be good for us if we could attain and maintain them. And of course the contrary is also true, specifically that it would be wrong, perhaps wicked, deliberately to put others in such a condition. Broadly speaking morality is about human flourishing. The good person will want to help others to flourish and to avoid thwarting their flourishing or destroying or damaging the conditions necessary for flourishing.[13]

There is of course a double moral analogue here of health and disability. That duality has what might be termed positive and negative aspects. The negative aspect is that the good reasons to avoid harm and disability, for ourselves and others, are moral reasons. They may also be prudential reasons, but these categories are not mutually exclusive. Just as it is wicked deliberately to harm others or to permit them to be harmed when we could reasonably have prevented it, it is wrongful to withhold rescue which we could reasonably perform—"Why didn't you warn me that the bridge had collapsed?"[14] The positive side of this coin is that where we can promote our own flourishing and the flourishing of others, we always have moral reasons so to do. Not of course necessarily moral

---

[12] Harris, *Enhancing Evolution*, Chapters 6 and 7.

[13] John Harris, "Is There a Coherent Social Conception of Disability?", *Journal of Medical Ethics*, vol. 26, no. 2 (2000): 95–101; John Harris, "One Principle and Three Fallacies of Disability Studies", *Journal of Medical Ethics*, vol. 27, no. 6 (2001): 383–8; John Harris, "One Principle and a Fourth Fallacy of Disability Studies", *Journal of Medical Ethics*, vol. 28, no. 3 (2002): 204.

[14] What "reasonably" means here I have discussed at length in *Violence and Responsibility*.

reasons "all things considered"—a point to which we will return in a moment. It is good to help others, bad to withhold the help that would spare them harm or suffering or promote flourishing and well-being. Good and bad in the moral sense of those terms. We may of course be entitled to abjure the good; rights and entitlements to do evil are not unknown; but I will not discuss them further now.

We understand very well what good and bad circumstances are and indeed generally how to avoid them for ourselves, and others. If we didn't we couldn't be prudent, we couldn't take care of ourselves, nor look out for others.

This is what the claim that the good is generic means and it is also how we argue for it. And there is a huge (although not of course total) consensus about what is good and bad for us; and again the existence of this consensus means that we know how to interpret the precautionary principle (with all its limitations) because we know what it is to be cautious and we know what it is to care.

The truism that we know how to take care of ourselves (and others) and indeed how to be prudent reminds us not only that we understand that good is generic but accept that it is.

A morally vital question is always "Why on earth did you hurt him?" or "How could you have let that terrible thing happen to her?" These questions are not simply a form of scolding, but a request for an appropriate moral justification in the knowledge that others will understand immediately why our conduct is in question here—because they understand how important it is that we preserve ourselves and others from harm. And that would be impossible to know or to teach without general agreement about what constitutes harm and benefit.

2.3 The Emergency Room Test

A test I have proposed for identifying what a disability or an injury or disease is, is the following, and the test has analogues for benefits:

Suppose a patient was admitted unconscious to the Accident and Emergency Department (the Emergency Room) of a hospital in a particular condition (no matter what it is at the moment) and the condition could be easily and immediately reversed, but not reversed unless the doctor acts without delay. If the condition is one that that doctor would be negligent were she not to attempt reversal then it is a disease, injury, or disability. I call this "the emergency room test".

Or, imagine a pregnant mother is made aware that a condition affects the child she is expecting; suppose further that the mother knows that the condition affecting her foetus could be removed permanently by a simple dietary adjustment? If the condition is in any way, however trivially, harmful to her potential child then surely, to fail to do so would be to knowingly harm her child. It will be clear that on this account of disability, disease, or "harmed condition", it would not be a disability, for example, to be born a Jew or a gipsy or black in Germany in the 1930s because whereas someone might well have a strong rational preference not to be in any of these 'conditions' in the stipulated circumstances, they are none of them in any sense "harmed conditions"; they do not harm the individual unless others cause that harm to the individual as a result of their being a person of the irrationally hated kind. In other words the harm is not intrinsic to the condition they are in but inflicted by others on the spurious ground that their existential state merits it. On the other hand, disabilities or diseases which adversely affect the functioning of the organism, are usually . . . well, dysfunctional.[15]

2.4 Human Flourishing and Human Rights

Longevity is an interesting test case. If and when strategies for vastly increasing life expectancy become available,[16] to be born with the possibility of living only a normal lifespan when others can live substantially longer, and when the individual in question could have been enabled to live longer, would count as being disabled to some degree because rational people would want the chance of a longer life (remember they don't have to accept that chance). Equally, if they were denied such a chance they would be left in a harmed condition relative to those with longer life expectancy. Short life expectancy or the opportunity to extend worthwhile life would surely meet the emergency room test.

---

[15] John Harris, "No Sex Selection Please, We're British!", *Journal of Medical Ethics*, vol. 31, no. 5 (2005): 286–8; John Harris, "Sex Selection and Regulated Hatred", *Journal of Medical Ethics*, vol. 31, no. 5 (2005): 291–4; John Harris, "Intimations of Immortality", *Science*, vol. 288, no. 5463 (2000): 59; Harris, "One Principle and Three Fallacies of Disability Studies"; Harris, *The Value of Life*.

[16] Harris, "Intimations of Immortality"; John Harris, "Intimations of Immortality: The Ethics and Justice of Life Extending Therapies", in Michael Freeman (ed.), *Current Legal Problems, Volume 55* (Oxford: Oxford University Press, 2002), pp. 65–97.

On this view a harmed condition is defined relative both to one's rational preferences and to conditions which might be described as harmful. Disability injury or harm are then to be understood, not relative to normal species functioning, but relative to possible alternatives. This is very important because so many of those who write about disabilities not only persist in the fallacious view that disability, impairment, or indeed illness must be defined relative to normal species functioning, or species typical functioning and seem unable to contemplate clear alternative accounts. Normal species functioning cannot form part of the definition of disability because people might be normal and still disabled in the sense that there are things they would want to do and cannot do that others can.

Suppose due to further depletions to the ozone layer, all white-skinned people were very vulnerable to skin cancers on even slight exposure to the sun, but brown- and black-skinned people were immune. We might then regard white people as suffering substantial disabilities relative to their darker-skinned fellows. And if skin pigmentation could be easily altered, failure to make the alterations would be injurious. We will return to the issue of enhancements later. For the moment it is sufficient to note that in such circumstances whites might have disabilities or deficits relative to blacks even though their functioning was quite species-typical or normal.

It is of course difficult to spell out exactly what one would and should call a "harmed condition". Harms can be quite slight but still be harms; and of course factors that harm the functioning of an organism can be in that organism's overall interests—if they could not, surgical procedures would never be indicated.[17]

Again it helps to apply the emergency room test. A harmed condition is one which, if a patient was brought unconscious into the Accident and Emergency Department of a hospital in such a condition and it could be reversed or removed then the medical staff would be negligent if they failed to reverse or remove it. So, for example, although the loss of the first joint of the little finger would be a small harm to bear, if someone came into hospital with the little finger severed at the first joint and it could be sewn on again, the staff would be negligent not to do so; they

---

[17] Harris, *Wonderwoman and Superman*, pp. 91–2.

would have harmed the patient by failing to restore the finger. Few would suggest that the loss of the tip of a little finger would make life unbearable or not worth living. That is not the point. The point is that any gratuitous harm is what it is, a gratuitous harm, and causing gratuitous harm is always unethical.

These points are crucial because it is sometimes said that while we have an obligation to cure disease—to restore normal functioning—we do not have an obligation to enhance or improve upon a normal healthy life, that enhancing function is permissive but could not be regarded as obligatory. But what constitutes a normal healthy life is determined in part by technological and medical and other advances (hygiene, sanitation, etc.). It is normal now, for example, to be protected against tetanus and polio; the continued provision of such protection is not merely permissive. If and when cheap and effective vaccines are developed for AIDS or malaria or Ebola, it would surely not be coherent to regard making available such preventive and therapeutic measures as permissive rather than mandatory. In most developed countries the tap water is drinkable. To allow this situation to lapse would be unethical as well as harmful.

It is also true that what health care providers regard as priorities for their service are no indication of the merits of available interventions or as to what people should be able to access if they choose. These issues have preoccupied me in other places over many years.[18] For example, human enhancement technologies and modalities which affect academic ability, or cognitive high performance more generally, sporting ability, or other dimensions of non-therapeutically relevant functioning, are often regarded as beyond the remit of health care provision. If and where this view holds, it is no evidence as to the importance or legitimacy of a moral distinction between therapy and enhancement (assuming such a distinction exists).[19]

This is not an exhaustive account of harm or benefit but it is a way of thinking about it that avoids certain obvious pitfalls. First, it does not define good or bad states of being in terms of any conception of normalcy. Second, it does not depend on post hoc ratification by the subject of the condition—it is not a prediction about how the subject of

---

[18] Harris, *Wonderwoman and Superman* and *Enhancing Evolution*.
[19] Harris, *Wonderwoman and Superman* and *Enhancing Evolution*.

the condition will feel. This is important because we need an account of disability and less specifically of harms and benefits we can use for the potentially self-conscious—gametes, embryos, foetuses, and neonates—and for the temporarily unconscious, which does not wait upon subsequent ratification by the person concerned.

Equally there is vast agreement about what conduces to human flourishing and to well-being. Often of course this is simply the absence of disease, disability, or other harms; but the positive side of flourishing, while perhaps slightly more problematic, still commands wide agreement. We value, in a way that makes the promotion of these things at least to some extent unproblematic, and in no special order: education, intelligence, leisure, adequate nourishment, good food, adequate housing and disposable income, a good (and rewarding) job, health, exercise, friends, family, love, sex (with or without the more controversial addition of drugs and rock 'n' roll), peace, (and quiet?), and preservation of the natural world, and indeed excitement. Personally we also usually value the virtues: courage, integrity, compassion, honesty, gentleness . . . and well . . . you get the picture! And to a certain extent I would expect also agreement as to how to rank order (roughly) the list for importance or urgency. We all have our own lists, but the overlap between all our lists will be vast. We know the good. Not maybe the whole good and certainly not nothing but the good, but without the help of God or the Gods we know enough about the good to value and promote it, to defend it and wish it to continue.

2.5 Justice and Human Rights

This is only very coincidentally a book about justice; but it is clear that absent a basis for discrimination, our moral imperatives to do good and prevent harm are imperatives that are impartial and apply to our relationships with all people. Moreover, justice, fairness, and equality are clearly also conditions necessary for human flourishing and injustice and inequity are harms as old and familiar as pain and suffering.

So morality is not problematic: it is doing good and preventing harm, to all—so far so quasi-analytic. But as I have just suggested, the further analysed nature of good and evil is (mostly) also unproblematic, commonplace, and widely shared among the human community, and we may predict also among our further evolved successors, the post-human community (and possibly also machine persons). If further evidence were needed we might note that the wide agreement about the nature and importance of what by some are called "human rights", and of the nature of those rights, strengthens our confidence in the fact that we do know what the minimum conditions for human flourishing are and how to promote them.

For the record I am not enthusiastic about the attempt to characterize the entitlements, interests, and mutual obligations of persons in terms of "rights". For traditional consequentialist reasons I judge that rights are always part of the conclusion of a moral argument and never one of its premises. Indeed, in legal and political discussions of human rights, such alleged rights usually function in a more nuanced sense as defeasible claims.[20] These issues are discussed further in the following chapter.

There are other good reasons for being critical of human rights as a way of framing entitlements for reasons that will appear in the course of this book, (especially Chapter 3). However, with caveats noted I think that human rights talk is here to stay, as long at least as there are still humans around who value it or to whom such talk seems appropriate. My point is that agreement, not about framing entitlements as rights, but agreement about the content of very important entitlements—the entitlement to, the right to, privacy and family life, free speech, a fair criminal trial, and so on—remains substantial.

Likewise the increasing international acceptance of the importance of ensuring wide access to health care and to essential medicines[21]

[20] John Harris, "Taking the 'Human' Out of Human Rights", *Cambridge Quarterly of Healthcare Ethics*, vol. 20, no. 1 (2010): 9–20, a version of which appears as the next chapter.

[21] *Who Owns Science: The Manchester Manifesto*: <http://www.isei.manchester.ac.uk/TheManchesterManifesto.pdf>.

Universal Declaration of Human Rights (1948 [cited 30 November 2010]): <http://www.ohchr.org/EN/UDHR/Documents/UDHR_Translations/eng.pdf>. Solomon R. Benatar, "Reflections and Recommendations on Research Ethics in Developing Countries", *Social Science & Medicine*, vol. 54, no. 7 (2002): 1131–41. World Health Organization, *Macroeconomics and Health: Investing in Health for Economic Development*. Report of the Commission on Macroeconomics and Health (Geneva: WHO, 2001). Joseph Stiglitz, "Scrooge and Intellectual Property Rights", *British Medical Journal*, vol. 333, no. 7582 (2006): 1279–80. Aidan Hollis and Thomas Pogge, *The Health Impact Fund: Making New Medicines Accessible for All* (Incentives for Global Health, 2008). UN Millennium Development Goals: Goal 8, "Develop a Global Partnership for Development". Target 8.E "In cooperation with pharmaceutical companies, provide access to affordable essential drugs in developing countries": <http://www.un.org/millenniumgoals/global.shtml>; WHO and the Office of the United Nations High Commissioner for Human Rights, June 2008, Factsheet

re-enforces my (and I hope your) confidence that the nature of the good is neither esoteric, nor inaccessible to us—quite the contrary!

2.6 Can Values be Objective?

And if all this sounds a bit G. E. Moore,[22] perhaps Moore was on to something. As Wittgenstein notes:[23]

> From its seeming to me—or to everyone—to be so, it doesn't follow that it is so. What we can ask is whether it can make sense to doubt it.[24]

When, later in the same place Wittgenstein observes "Knowledge is in the end based on acknowledgement"[25] I believe he is making a point importantly related to the one I am trying to make here; namely that our acceptance of the importance of human rights, of provision of health care and social welfare, in short of the familiar and generic nature of what is good and bad for people like us, constitutes our acknowledgement of the fact that we well know all this, and know it in an appropriate use of the concept of knowledge.

> The difference between the concept of 'knowing' and the concept of 'being certain' isn't of any great importance at all, except where "I know" is meant to mean: I *can't* be wrong.[26]

The class of things about which "I can't be wrong" may be infinite (there are for example an infinite number of things that are true by definition) but that is not significant. So, we know what's good for us and what's bad for us. But how reliably?

No. 31, "The Right to Health": <http://www.who.int/hhr/activities/Right_to_Health_fac tsheet31.pdf>. WHO, "Access to essential medicines as part of the human right to health": <http://www.who.int/medicines/areas/human_rights/en/>. *Health and Human Rights Journal*, vol. 15, no. 2 (2013), 1–4: "The Post-2015 Development Agenda", Human Rights, Evidence and Open-Access Publishing: <http://www.hhrjournal.org/wp-content/uploads/sites/13/2013/12/Editorial-The-post-2015-development-agenda-human-rights-evidence-and-open-access-publishing-.pdf>.

[22] <http://plato.stanford.edu/entries/moore/>, accessed 16 January 2014.

[23] G. E. Moore, "Proof of an External World", *Proceedings of the British Academy*, vol. 25 (1939): 273–300; Ludwig Wittgenstein, *On Certainty*, ed. G. E. M. Anscombe and G. H. Von Wright (Oxford: Basil Blackwell, 1969), para. 1, p. 2e.

[24] Wittgenstein, *On Certainty*, para. 2.   [25] Wittgenstein, *On Certainty*, para. 379.

[26] Wittgenstein, *On Certainty*, para. 8.

We are all too familiar with the history of what we might call moral blindness, the human habit of excluding candidates for full moral status, "personhood" as I would call it.[27] This has happened to/with outsiders of various sorts: people from other families, clans, villages, and societies and equally to people within those groups or societies: women, children, slaves, peasants, and people of different race, skin-colour, and social class. We have been dreadfully, wickedly, wrong about all of these people; judging them inferior, or to be inappropriate objects of our full moral concern (but not of course all of us all of the time). Moral knowledge like all other forms of knowledge has developed over time, and the history of science, as well as of sensibility, is littered with mistakes and is, one might say, often characterized by an inability to see or interpret what is present to our senses. The mistakes are identified only by a combination of evidence and argument, by rationality if you like. We may feel (have felt) that there is/was something wrong with excluding women from civil rights, rights like the franchise and from the demands of justice, such as equal pay for equal work; but the discrimination is eventually revealed as prejudice, there being demonstrably no relevant basis for prejudicial discrimination. There is simply no relevant difference between women and men that might justify different treatment in matters of rights justice and opportunity. Indeed we humans still find overbearingly strong purchase in the perceived differences in moral obligations owed by persons of different states, one to another, and this leads to enormous, avoidable harm.

When I use the inclusive term "we" here, for example when pointing to examples of moral progress, I am of course aware that such progress is not currently either universally accepted or expressed, and may apply primarily to liberal democracies, and to non-theocratic states. Science is none the less objective despite the fact that there are millions of people in the world who do not accept Darwinian evolution and who reject climate change.

Gains in knowledge are incremental and cumulative, and one breakthrough leads to another, as with science. Once made, the gains seem solid. We are not (if we know what's good for us, and we do) going back to Ptolemaic cosmology and we are not going back to societies built on slavery or to white or male supremacy. Which is not of course to say that

---

[27] Harris, *Violence and Responsibility*, Chapter 1; Harris, *The Value of Life*, Chapter 1; Harris, "The Concept of the Person and the Value of Life"; Harris, "Taking the 'Human' Out of Human Rights".

either slavery or male supremacy have, as yet, been entirely eradicated. They have, however, been comprehensively morally discredited. I hope it is clear that from the fact that some values are matters of knowledge, of fact if you like, it does not follow that all are, nor does it follow that all could be.

I would venture a guess (but it is only a guess, since I have not attempted to catalogue the moral mistakes of the past, nor those we are still making),[28] that most of our real howlers have been mistakes of exclusion, however motivated. We have excluded from moral consideration individuals and classes of being that should not have been excluded. The only way to identify these sorts of mistake is to explore carefully the grounds, the reasons, and purported justifications for including or excluding individuals from types of moral consideration, and to constantly review those decisions. The defence of this idea is the business of this book. We may be making our biggest mistake yet, that mistake exemplified by the idea of human rights,[29] namely that there is something special about species membership, which confers rights, or grounds interests. This issue will be the subject of the next chapter.

2.7 Our Evolutionary Limitations

It is important also to bear in mind that there may be levels of altruism that cannot be reached by we ape-descended creatures, with our evolutionary story so far. Both utopian morality and utopian politics may be blighted by the limitations imposed by our evolved moral psychology and its possible roots in primitive pro-social behaviour; more of which anon. There are also, as Martin Rees has observed, probably related limitations on science. There may be scientific facts that will never be discovered by beings with brains that have evolved in the way that human brains have so far developed, and scientific theories we are incapable of postulating.[30] There may be differences between these two sets of limitations. Martin Rees, I think, had in mind ideas or possibilities that are literally unthinkable to people with minds like ours. The moral possibilities to which I have alluded

---

[28] See Jonathan Glover, *Humanity: A Moral History of the Twentieth Century* (London: Jonathan Cape, 1999).

[29] Harris, "Taking the 'Human' Out of Human Rights".

[30] <http://www.ox.ac.uk/media/news_stories/2011/111103_1.html>, accessed 17 January 2014; *The Sunday Times*, London, 13 June 2010.

are obviously not unthinkable; more probably, and possibly more simply, they may be undoable by people, or by all but a very few people, at our current evolutionary stage.

2.8 The Social Contract is Not Just a Theory of Government

The limitations of individual morality do not necessarily, however, apply collectively. The obligations we may owe to one another seem sometimes overwhelming, particularly when they are seen as involving negative responsibility (our responsibility for the consequences of omissions) as well as positive responsibility (our responsibility for the consequences of doings rather than simply of refrainings).[31] Mutual moral responsibilities may, however, be more realistic and achievable at a society or national level by such beings as are we, than they are at the individual level. Public services are a good example. Health, welfare, and national defence are unlikely to be effectively deliverable in modern societies by individual action or private initiatives. So that levels of altruism that are beyond the power of individuals may be effectively deliverable by governments or other social institutions. No individual can usually hope to "feed the poor", defend the weak, or "heal the sick", but good social welfare and health services and infrastructure (whether publicly or privately funded) can and do so far as this is possible at all. I discuss state or collective responsibility and its grounds in more detail in Chapter 11.

While public assumption of responsibility for health and welfare and indeed the delivery of the required services are usually, if not the prerogative, certainly the business of nation states there are some private initiatives on some aspects of health and welfare of commensurate scale: for example, those of the Bill and Melinda Gates Foundation (supported by Warren Buffett) and funders supporting health research such as the Wellcome Trust.[32] However, while wonderful additions to health welfare provision for many and virtually the only source of such provision for many more it is noteworthy that private agencies are not accountable to

---

[31] I wrote about acts and omissions extensively in my book *Violence and Responsibility*.
[32] <http://www.gatesfoundation.org/What-We-Do>; <http://www.wellcome.ac.uk/index. htm>, accessed 22 January 2014.

the people they help (except perhaps through their own rules, the law of negligence, and other applicable national legislation).

The only problem left is to work out how effectively to secure the good for ourselves and others and to ensure that the relevant others are properly identified. (The others to which I refer are other persons, not necessarily other human beings. There may be other candidates for full inclusion but as yet I am unconvinced of their merits. The arguments for this and the inclusions and exclusions which those arguments justify, I have detailed elsewhere.)[33] The only reliable and safe method of attempting to determine who matters morally, and how much they matter, is by reflection on what confers moral status and why.[34]

The only way of determining what we should do by way of moral enhancement is to rationally consider the various ways of securing the good and preventing harm, and getting better at spotting potential dangers, like climate change, and acting quickly enough, where effective strategies are available, to prevent their worst effects.

2.9 Anti-Philosophy

I have suggested that in order to be as confident as we can be of the moral success of our deeds we need to know, or rather believe, more than that these actions are well motivated. Indeed, for these purposes, we do not even need to know whether or not they are well motivated. What we need above all is to know they are for the best, all things considered.

A philosopher notorious for trying to do away with moral philosophy and rely directly on feelings is Leon Kass. Talking about cloning he says:

We are repelled by the prospect of cloning human beings not because of the strangeness or novelty of the undertaking, but because we intuit and feel, immediately and without argument, the violation of things that we rightfully hold dear.[35]

The problem that confronts Kass, and anyone who wishes to cut to the chase of morality by finding ways to decide or to act "immediately and without argument" is to have a way of knowing when one's sense of outrage, or one's "feelings" or whatever, are evidence of something

---

[33] Harris, *Violence and Responsibility*.   [34] Harris, *The Value of Life*.
[35] Leon R. Kass, "The Wisdom of Repugnance", *The New Republic* (2 June 1997): 17–26. I discuss Kass's approach in *Enhancing Evolution*, Chapter 8.

morally disturbing and when they are simply an expression of bare prejudice or simply an induced emotional response. George Orwell,[36] as I fondly recall, referred to this reliance on intuition or emotion as the use of "moral nose"; as if one could simply sniff a situation and smell or feel the rightness or wrongness. The problem is that nasal reasoning is notoriously unreliable and difficult to assess objectively, and olfactory ethics, despite being widely practised, has never really taken off as an academic discipline.[37] Despite this lack of a theoretical base, so to speak, olfactory moral philosophy has many contemporary adherents.

Kass, for example, in disarmingly admitting that revulsion "is not an argument", seems to be implying the existence of some other way of determining that the revulsion is "rightfully" felt.[38] But how can he know this without having either evidence or argument to explain how the feelings are somehow "rightful"? The term "rightfully" implies a judgement or some other supporting evidence which confirms the veracity of the claim he is making. If it is simply one feeling confirming another, then we really are in the situation Wittgenstein lampooned as buying a second copy of the same newspaper to confirm the truth of what we read in the first.[39] As Wittgenstein, albeit emphasizing the obvious, insisted: "justification consists in appealing to something independent".[40]

2.10 Why Do We Need to Appeal to Something Independent?

As I have argued elsewhere,[41] someone who cares about doing the right thing, someone for whom the difference between right and wrong is

---

[36] In a letter to Humphrey House, 11 April 1940: *The Collected Essays, Journalism and Letters of George Orwell*, vol. 1 (Harmondsworth: Penguin, 1970), p. 583. See my more detailed discussion of the problems with this type of reasoning in *Wonderwoman and Superman*, Chapter 2, and in my *Violence and Responsibility*, p. 112. Orwell's idea has been taken up by others. See H. A. Chapman, D. A. Kim, J. M. Susskind, and A. K. Anderson, "In Bad Taste: Evidence for the Oral Origins of Moral Disgust", *Science*, vol. 323, no. 5918 (2009): 1222–6.

[37] I first outlined the basics of olfactory ethics in my book *Violence and Responsibility*, pp. 111ff.

[38] Here the argument follows lines taken in Harris, *Enhancing Evolution*, pp. 129 ff.

[39] Ludwig Wittgenstein, *Philosophical Investigations*, trans. G. E. M. Anscombe, 3rd edn. (Oxford: Basil Blackwell, 2001), para. 265, p. 79e.

[40] Wittgenstein, *Philosophical Investigations*, para. 265, p. 79e.

[41] *Inter alia* and most recently in John Harris, "'Ethics is for Bad Guys!': Putting the 'Moral' into Moral Enhancement", *Bioethics*, vol. 27, no. 3 (2013): 169–73.

important, will always want to ask him or herself if what feels right is right. They will want to assure themselves that insofar as it is in their power, they really are acting well or for the best all things considered, that what seems right is right. They will, in short, be interested in a crucial distinction, emphasized by no less a reflective thinking being than Hamlet himself, in this famous riposte to his mother: "Seems, madam? Nay it is. I know not 'seems'."[42] The difference between what seems and what is in ethics can only be delivered by reasoning.

There is a rather different argument, familiar to philosophers and indeed to theologians.[43] It derives from Plato[44] and has been used by Kant and many others. It sets out a different way of thinking about one of the central points of my argument against moral enhancement, understood as the manipulation of pro-social responses. This argument is directed to establishing the independent, essentially analytic nature of morality.

In Plato's dialogue known as "Euthyphro", Socrates is educating Euthyphro about holiness:

But, friend Euthyphro, if that which is holy were the same with that which is dear to the gods, and were loved because it is holy, then that which is dear to the gods would be loved as being dear to them; but if that which is dear to them were dear to them because loved by them, then that which is holy would be holy because loved by them. But now you see that the reverse is the case, and that the two things are quite different from one another. For one . . . is of a kind to be loved because it is loved, and the other . . . is loved because it is of a kind to be loved.

Bertrand Russell puts this argument rather more clearly to a twenty-first century ear.

[I]f you are quite sure that there is a difference between right and wrong then you are in this situation: is that difference due to God's fiat or is it not? If it is due to God's fiat, then for God Himself there is no difference between right and wrong, and it is no longer a significant statement to say that God is good. If you are going to say, as theologians do, that God is good, you must then say that right and wrong have some meaning, which is independent of God's fiat. Because God's fiats are good and not bad independently of the mere fact that He made them. If

---

[42]   William Shakespeare, *Hamlet*, Act 1, Scene 2, Arden Shakespeare.

[43]   See for example Anthony Kenny, *A Brief History of Western Philosophy* (Oxford: Basil Blackwell, 1998), pp. 25ff. and his "Afterword", pp. 346ff.

[44]   Plato, *The Dialogues*, 4th edn., trans. B. Jowett (Oxford: Clarendon Press, 1953), vol. 1, "Euthyphro", 10–11.

you are going to say that then you will have to say that it is not only through God that right and wrong came into being, but that they are in their essence logically anterior to God.[45]

This argument does not of course say anything about the existence of God, nor does it deny God's goodness. It merely points out that the statements "God is good" and "God is God" must have different meanings, if "good" is to have any meaning at all. One of God's great claims to fame, indeed to goodness, is that she wills the good. As Tony Kenny[46] puts the point: "even if . . . being loved by the gods is only something that happens to what is holy: it does not tell us the essential nature of holiness itself". Knowing that the gods love something does not tell us why they love it, why it ought to be loved. Being aware of the objects of our sympathetic attention tells us nothing about whether or not our sympathy or pro-sociality is appropriate or misplaced.

It is our ability to reason about the nature of the good independently of God's "fiat" as Russell calls it, or of knowledge about what the gods love, that partially accounts for theology and indeed enables us to say non-vacuously that God is, or that the gods are, good. For if we believe that gods only will the good, then if we can establish what is good, we have reason to choose between rival interpretations of the will of the gods. This is the problem we have when asking ourselves the question "Is what I seem drawn to do, is what my sympathies or my 'fellow feeling' prompt me to do, really what I should be doing; is it what's best?"

In John Locke's famous characterization of the proper use of the term person we see further reasons why.

We must consider what person stands for; which I think is a thinking intelligent being, that has reason and reflection, and can consider itself the same thinking thing, in different times and places; which it does only by that consciousness which is inseparable from thinking and seems to me essential to it; it being impossible for anyone to perceive without perceiving that he does perceive.[47]

[45] Bertrand Russell, "Why I Am Not a Christian", in *Why I Am Not a Christian and Other Essays* (London: George Allen & Unwin, 1957).

[46] Kenny, *Brief History*, pp. 27–8.

[47] John Locke, *An Essay Concerning Human Understanding*, ed. A. S. Pringle-Pattison (Oxford: Clarendon Press, 1964), Book II, Ch. 27. Locke formulated this definition in the middle of the seventeenth century.

2.11 What Do We Stand For?

When Locke speaks here of what "person stands for" he is talking, as he says, "forensically", he is recommending a considered description or definition. However, the word "person" stands for something in a different sense. We persons stand for a type of being which possibly exists nowhere else in the universe, a being capable of reason and reflection and hence also capable of considering the nature and quality of its acts, motives, and emotions with the ability to choose whether or not to act on the results of that deliberative process. In short we are creatures demonstrably capable of developing a moral outlook.

We persons stand for something important. First, we stand up to be counted or rather to be accountable. Accountable as beings with free will and hence as beings with a choice and hence beings who bear responsibility for the choices we make and for their consequences. We are the sorts of beings that can and do determine not only our own fate but the fate of others, and the state of the world we inhabit. We are creatures who are aware of the fact that this is what we are doing. With this power comes responsibility, and with the ability to reason and reflect comes the opportunity and the imperative to act on the results of that reasoning and reflective process.

Our capacities thus enable us usually to distinguish between good and bad (there are of course grey areas where we don't know what to say just as in science), and with the capacity to recognize these qualities come opportunities and responsibilities, to act to enhance the good and diminish the bad. And because of this we stand for decency and goodness; or rather we stand out as the only creatures so far identified who have any sense at all of decency and goodness, in short who have a morality properly so called.

These powers and capacities enable us to consider the differences between ourselves and other creatures and to ask ourselves about the extent to which such differences as we perceive justify or necessitate differences in the concern, respect, and protection we accord to those others and demand for ourselves.

The results of this highly deliberative process have been the emergence, and constant re-evaluation and refinement of moral and political principles, including principles of human rights and of justice, and the development of social and political institutions embodying these. The present point is that our long process of evolution and development has resulted in the emergence and flourishing of a system of personal and public morality which includes human rights. This system, whatever its evolutionary origins, is essentially and inherently deliberative and indeed depends, and has always depended on, a constant process of reason and reflection for its development, adjustment, and modification or reform for its continuation and all of these for whatever confidence people repose in it.[48] Indeed the modern political and social institutions that are the current culmination (but not we may hope an endpoint) of that process of development. Most democratic states depend upon the regular endorsement of their legitimacy in the form of the expressed consent of the governed. That is by the submission of themselves, their policies, and political and legal acts for the appraisal and consent of the electorate.

The seeking of that consent and approval in most cases takes the form of an argument, perhaps in the form of a political manifesto, written or not, to the effect that both what they have done in the past and propose for the future either conduces to the public good and indeed to the individual benefit of the electors; or at least that it is not manifestly contrary to the public good or the personal interests of the electorate broadly conceived.

Nothing that today can pass for morality or moral principles or precepts, can be isolated from reason and reflection on their adequacy, success, and effect just as nothing that today can pass for a defensible legislative and regulatory programme can be isolated from reason and reflection on the adequacy, success, and effect of that programme. Moreover, as I have argued in brief earlier, no one who claims to be acting morally or out of moral conviction or principle can resist accountability for what they claim to believe or do in the name of morality. Equally, no political party, whether in government or not, and claiming to be acting out of political conviction or principle can resist accountability for what they claim to believe or do in the name of the people. And this means they must always be prepared to offer a reasoned defence and justification of their morality or elements of it. It would never be

---

[48] Ray Tallis makes this point at some length and brilliantly in a number of places, particularly in his recent book *Aping Mankind: Neuromania, Darwinitis and the Misrepresentation of Humanity* (Durham: Acumen, 2011).

enough or indeed even respectable (in either morality or politics) for the reply to be "I just felt like it."[49]

Staying more strictly with morality for the moment, feeling is not enough but isn't it plausible to think with David Hume, that "morality is better felt than judged of"?

There is a distinction that can help here and that is the distinction between doing good and acting morally, between judgements about things that are ethically significant and ethical judgements. Not all judgements about things that are ethically important are ethical judgements. To be an ethical judgement rather than simply a judgement about something of ethical importance that judgement first has actually to be a *judgement*, not simply a pronouncement. A judgement moreover is a conclusion arrived at by a deliberative process, a process that involves the exercise of judgement. To count as a moral judgement that deliberative process of which it is part has to weigh alternatives from some justifiably moral perspective. For example it has to consider alternatives from the perspective of the amount and quality of the good that might thereby be achieved, or the rights that might thereby be protected or the justice that might thereby be done or the suffering that might be mitigated or avoided or by the number of lives saved or lost.

Just as a moral judgement is more than a statement that has some moral relevance, an argument is more than a series of contradictory statements. I am reminded of the famous "Monty Python" Argument Sketch about whether an argument consists of more than just contradiction. Does a judgement consist of more than just a statement and a moral act of more than an act with good consequences? Here is a fragment of the Python argument about argument. The man responds to a notice offering arguments at a price:

MAN: I came here for a good argument!
ARGUER: Ah no you didn't, you came here for an argument.
M: An argument isn't just contradiction.
A: Well! it CAN be!
M: No it can't.

---

[49] Ronald Dworkin elaborated this requirement for detailed and theory-based justification for moral claims in his *Taking Rights Seriously* (London: Duckworth, 1977), especially Chapters 7 and 8.

M: An argument is a connected series of statements intended to establish a proposition.

A: No it isn't.

M: Yes it is! 'tisn't just contradiction.

A: Look if I "argue" with you, I must take up a contrary position!

M: Yes but it isn't just saying 'no it isn't'.

A: Yes it is!

M: No it isn't![50]

I think the consensus is that the man who paid for an argument in the Python sketch was being short changed (though not the audience of course) and that just as an argument is more than just contradiction, a moral judgement is more than just a statement about something of moral relevance.

2.12 One Can Do Good Accidentally but One Cannot be Moral Accidentally

One can accidentally discover something of scientific importance but one cannot be scientific, one cannot do science, accidentally. Doing science is a deliberative and disciplined process, it involves for example doing things like formulating and testing a hypothesis, looking for disconfirmatory evidence as well as for confirmatory evidence; it is not simply finding white swans but looking for black ones. And looking for black ones for the purpose of testing the hypothesis. Simply finding a black swan is not "scientific behaviour" any more than finding a black swan necessarily tests the hypothesis that all swans are white; it is not necessarily even proto-scientific behaviour. The same goes analogously for moral behaviour.

Being moral is like being scientific. Hamlet again:

POLONIUS [aside] Though this be madness, yet there is
method in't. – Will you walk out of the air, my lord?
HAMLET Into my grave?
POLONIUS Indeed, that's out of the air.[51]

---

[50] From "Monty Python's Previous Record" and "Monty Python's Instant Record Collection".

[51] Shakespeare, *Hamlet*, Act 2, Scene 2.

This is a wonderful fragment about the scope and limits of scientific method. Polonius respects method but Hamlet uses a different methodology to confound him. Whether inviting someone to "walk out of the air" is remotely moral depends upon the reasons and justifications for so doing, the rational calculation of the probable results and the context in which it is done, not to say the resolution of some of the ambiguities inherent in language.

It should now be clear that not all behaviour, and not even all behaviour that affects moral outcomes, is moral behaviour any more than all behaviour that affects political outcomes is political behaviour. The relatively recent riots and looting in British cities clearly exhibits behaviour with profound moral and political consequences, but to call it moral or political behaviour is quite another thing. It could be both, but only if a particular, and a particularly complex and interesting, story accompanies the claim.

2.13 Moral Behaviour and Good People

There is a long-standing distinction in moral philosophy between judging persons and judging actions. This is necessary, not least because good people can do bad things and bad people can do good things. This distinction has even penetrated to the United Kingdom secret intelligence service. Dame Eliza Manningham-Buller, former Director General of MI5, said in her 2011 Reith Lecture: "Not all terrorists are evil though, their acts are."[52]

We thus need a moral sensibility capable of evaluating both the goodness of deeds and of their effects, in short of outcomes (consequentialism) and the goodness of people and their states of mind and dispositions (virtue ethics). If we are interested in the individual biography, we are interested, morally speaking, primarily in their virtues and vices. If we are interested in making the world a better place, we are interested in outcomes—consequences. Since most of us are more interested in what happens to us than the state of the soul of those who influence what happens to us, we tend to be for all practical purposes consequentialists. This is because even if we are not consequentialists and are interested in

[52] Eliza Manningham-Buller, Reith Lecture, BBC Radio 4, 20 September 2011.

virtues and our state of mind (or of grace) we need to be confident we will have the freedom to develop our virtues according to our own values and this requires that others leave us that free space. Hence whatever the state of their souls we need them to leave us free to cultivate our own in ways that we find virtuous.

To put this point another way, it is easier and safer (for what both want) for consequentialists to neglect virtues than for virtue ethicists to neglect consequences.

This is why moral behaviour cannot simply be a matter of moral emotions or states of mind or intentions or even brain states. Good intentions or emotions or states of mind, without the careful and realistic calculation of consequence, without, in short considering if not all things, at least as many possible consequences of conduct as time allows and appear relevant, is a recipe not only for disaster but for the triumph of evil. To be good, "thank you very much!" is then to act for the best all things considered. To prioritize the avoidance of, for example, so-called direct harms, is neither the action of a good conscience, nor that of a good consequentialist.

We now turn progressively to issues of how we can improve morality, in short how we can make the world a better place. And hence how we know when someone is good, when they are acting well. But first in the next chapter we turn to some further thoughts upon how our species, human beings, indeed on the extent to which being human, matters.

3

Taking the Human out of Human Rights

Moral enhancement like many other enhancing methodologies is changing human nature, hopefully, if these methodologies are well conceived, changing human nature and eventually humanity itself for the better.[1] These changes may eventually lead to the further evolution of our species to the extent of its replacement by a successor species. We have noted that attempts to be and do good involve identifying, deciding, and acting for the best all things considered. Such action may be individual or collective and much turns on policies decided on, or adopted and implemented by governments nationally and internationally. One mechanism for attempting to ensure that vital interests are protected and hence that moral standards are upheld is the concept of human rights and the mechanisms whereby such rights are understood and interpreted, promoted, and upheld. Such mechanisms have done and continue to do a power of good in the world. However, they may be misconceived in one very important respect which involves a possibly self-defeating parochialism. In this chapter we examine why this is and how its dangerous consequences might be avoided.

Human rights are universally acknowledged to be important, although they are of course by no means universally respected. This universality has helped to combat racism and sexism and other arbitrary and vicious forms of discrimination. Unfortunately, as we shall see, the universality

[1] Work on this chapter reflects my collaboration with John Sulston on many of the themes here developed. I have also benefited from comments by John Coggon, Sarah Chan, and Annabelle Lever on earlier drafts of this material. An earlier version of this chapter was published as: John Harris, "Taking the 'Human' out of Human Rights", *The Cambridge Quarterly of Healthcare Ethics*, vol. 20, no. 1 (2010): 9–20.

of human rights is both too universal and not universal enough.[2] It is time to take the "human" out of human rights.[3] Indeed, it is very probable, as we have noted, that in the future there will be no more humans as we know them now, since the further evolution of our species, either Darwinian, or more likely determined by human choices,[4] will, we must hope, result in the emergence of new sorts of beings better able to cope with the intellectual and physical challenges of the future. One example of the ways in which this is already happening is the sorts of cognitive enhancement that are already coming on stream;[5] another has been long signalled by stem cell research and the birth and flourishing of regenerative medicine.

Human rights are one of the most important and universally accepted ideas both in moral and political philosophy and in contemporary jurisprudence. While appeals to human rights are by no means unproblematic, where there is agreement or jurisprudential support for the existence of particular human rights this fact becomes a powerful tool for the protection of such rights and for the remedies that such protection affords. It is a pity then that the insertion of "human" into human rights has occurred so thoughtlessly and with such little attention to the prejudice of which this is an expression and to the extent to which this terminology may make future generations of beings like us, hostages to fortune. In this chapter we explore the desirability and the consequences of separating human rights from human nature in the sense of species membership but significantly not from other aspects of our evolved nature. We noted in Chapter 2 the ways in which morality is connected to what constitutes benefits and harms to creatures like us; in the final chapter of this book we return to the ways in which our morality may be rooted, if not in human nature, then in aspects of that nature which

---

[2] Too universal because there are many humans to which it cannot and does not apply (see John Harris, *The Value of Life* (London: Routledge, 1985)) and not universal enough for reasons also examined in that book and, *inter alia*, in my *Enhancing Evolution* (Princeton and Oxford: Princeton University Press, 2007).

[3] And indeed the "dignity" out of human dignity. Analogous arguments show that the concept of human dignity is equally vacuous and redundant. See also Ruth Macklin, "Dignity is a Useless Concept", *BMJ*, vol. 327, no. 7429 (2003): 1419–20.

[4] Harris, *Enhancing Evolution*.

[5] Henry Greely, Barbara Sahakian, John Harris, Ron Kessler, Michael Gazzaniga, Philip Campbell, and Martha Farah, "Towards Responsible Use of Cognitive Enhancing Drugs by the Healthy", *Nature*, vol. 456, no. 7223 (2008): 702–5.

enable us to understand what is good and bad for us and hence how to further our own interests and the interests of other beings relevantly like us. Here we look at the ways in which the concept of human rights has promoted a culture which has inflated the importance of being human, in ways that may prevent us from seeing the moral significance of other sorts of beings.

Joseph Raz has commented, the "traditional approach" takes "human rights to be those important rights which are grounded in our humanity.[6] The underlying thought is that the arguments which establish that a putative right-holder has a human right rely on no *contingent* fact except laws of nature, the nature of humanity and that the right holder is a human being."[7] In an illuminating footnote Raz comments "One may allow that permanently comatose people do not have human rights. But one abandons the idea that human rights derive from our humanity once one says that babies or people with Down Syndrome do not have (certain) human rights." Raz goes on to advance a positive account of human rights identifying them as those rights "regarding which sovereignty measures are morally justified" by which he means rights which "set limits to the sovereignty of states".[8] However, Raz does not seriously consider non-human or partially human candidates for human rights however defined[9] and the question remains as to what or who are the rights-holders over which limits are set to the sovereignty of states.

A deep question, and one begged by the traditional accounts of human rights just noted, is: what role does "humanity", species membership, being a human being, in short the descriptive sense of being human, play in our evaluative use of that term? When we identify humanity not simply with species membership, being a human being, but with being

---

[6] For examples of this traditional approach see James Nickel, *Making Sense of Human Rights* (Oxford: Blackwell, 2006), p. 38; John Tasioulas, "The Moral Reality of Human Rights", in Thomas Pogge (ed.), *Freedom from Poverty as a Human Right* (Oxford: Oxford University Press, 2007), pp. 75–103; Alan Gewirth, *Human Rights: Essays on Justifications and Applications* (Chicago: University of Chicago Press, 1982), p. 41 and Peter Jones, "Human Rights", in the *Routledge Encyclopedia of Philosophy*, ed. Edward Craig: <http://www.rep.routledge.com/article/S105>.

[7] Joseph Raz, "Human Rights Without Foundations", in S. Besson and J. Tasioulas (eds.), *The Philosophy of International Law* (Oxford: Oxford University Press, 2010), pp. 321–38.

[8] Raz, "Human Rights Without Foundations", pp. 12 and 11 respectively (online version).

[9] Although Raz's account is consistent with the one developed in this chapter.

a moral being we may be claiming one of two very different things. The first is that we humans, the species *Homo sapiens sapiens*, are characterized by, among other qualities, moral agency and other important features like the capacities for sympathy, empathy, and creativity. The second implies more: that the possession of these qualities is essentially human, possessed by us only because we are the species that we are. This second sense implies that our humanity in the moral sense is not simply species typical, but rather it requires being human in the biological or genetic sense. There is not only a danger, there is a long-established and deeply ingrained habit and tradition of identifying properties or qualities that are contingently possessed by human beings as necessarily possessed by our kind and, moreover, necessarily not possessed by other kinds.

When we ask questions like "what is it to be human?", or talk about a person's "humanity" or talk of the "human spirit" or "human values", we not only emphasize the properties that typically distinguish our species from species not capable of having values, we indulge in a sort of chauvinism, celebrating our own kind as we do in a different sense when we talk of "Britishness", "European Culture", or "Western Civilization".[10]

This human chauvinism is often given a pseudo-scientific bent which is inimical to both the spirit of science and indeed to free inquiry. There is often talk of "species barriers"[11] as if, insofar as such things exist, they are laws of nature set up not simply to protect our supposed species purity, but to preserve those qualities we possess that may not only be currently particularly strongly represented in, or typical of, our species but may be unique to this planet. Of course we should not lose these properties but the question is should we improve upon them if we can? And a further important question is: should we restrict these properties to our own species?

---

[10] Gandhi was once asked, allegedly by a reporter, what he thought of Western Civilization. He replied that he thought "it would be a very good thing". I believe this was after a tour of London but I have been unable to find an authoritative source. <http://en.wikiquote.org/wiki/Gandhi>.

[11] The idea of species barriers I have criticized in John Harris, "Transhumanity: A Moral Vision of the Twenty-First Century", in N. Ann Davis, Richard Keshen, and Jeff McMahan (eds.), *Ethics and Humanity: Themes from the Philosophy of Jonathan Glover* (New York: Oxford University Press, 2009), pp. 155–72.

We do not want to lose our essential humanity if by that is meant those "human" characteristics that we value; but could we have not only those characteristics but also improve upon them if that is possible and add others that we do or would value to an equal or greater extent?

A number of recent developments in biotechnology and in our understanding of evolution indicate that the time has come not only for a reassessment of the role of "human" in human rights but of the idea of "humanity" in our conceptions of ourselves and of our place and our future in the universe. We will consider some of these before drawing some conclusions about the future of our species and the rights we have arrogated to ourselves.

3.1 Humanimals

Creatures with human and animal features are perennially fascinating; two of the most familiar and frequently mentioned examples are centaurs and mermaids but there are many others and science fiction continues to provide new examples.[12]

I prefer to use the term "humanimal" to cover any biological entities, whether individual creatures or cells, which have any mixture of animal and human elements.

Humanimals have been created for many years, and hybrids have almost certainly always existed naturally; however, the ethics of their creation and use is still in its infancy. A recent report by the United Kingdom Academy of Medical Sciences (AMS)[13] identifies many aspects of basic science that have been and continue to be studied in ways which involve the "mixing" of animal and human derived cells, in particular "understanding the nature and potential of stem cells"—one of the most promising avenues of therapeutic and basic research that involves the study of the behaviour of these cells in animal models, including of course human as well as animal derived stem cells. As the AMS report notes, "there are thousands of examples of transgenic animals, mostly

---

[12] In this section I borrow from my "Transhumanity: A Moral Vision of the Twenty-First Century".

[13] *Inter-Species Embryos: A Report by the Academy of Medical Sciences* (June 2007; ISBN 1–903401–15–1). The present author acknowledges his co-authorship of this report and thanks fellow members of the Academy Working Group for many useful insights.

mice, containing human DNA, mainly used as models of human gene function and human disease".[14] The report notes that approaches "involving 'secondary' chimeras, i.e. the transfer of human cells into animals at a later stage of development, are already in widespread use in studies of human and mouse pluripotent and tissue-specific stem cells". It is also common practice to "investigate the potential of human neural stem cells to integrate appropriately into mouse or rat brain as a test of their potential safety and usefulness".[15] Such interspecies humanimal research is widespread and is required not only for basic science but to develop and prove applications designed to treat serious human disease. As with all research at its outset, long-term and established benefits are necessarily in the future.[16]

The ethical question is whether the sanctity of so-called species barriers, or other objections to interspecies constructs affords good or even plausible reasons to abandon such research and forgo or postpone whatever benefits it might yield. The deeper theoretical and perhaps political question is whether interspecies creatures or enhanced human creatures created not by mixing matter from different species but by engineering further evolution or admixing or interfacing non-organic technical elements with human biology might not only create better sorts of creatures but whether such combinations have any necessary or for that matter contingent connection with the rights and responsibilities such creatures might have. Before further addressing this question we must remind ourselves of some assumptions and attitudes we have inherited.

3.2 The Mermaid Myth

It is important to distinguish between the creation of a human embryo incorporating animal material that will not be allowed to develop further, and the possibility of bringing such an embryo to term so that it will become a living independent creature. In the case of the embryo what will be created will simply be cells that will be maintained solely in vitro,

---

[14] *Inter-Species Embryos*, p. 3 and p. 33.

[15] *Inter-Species Embryos*, p. 34. See Olle Linvall and Zaal Kokala, "Stem Cells for the Treatment of Neurological Disorders", *Nature*, vol. 441, no. 7097 (2006): 1094–6.

[16] As of course are so-called "adverse effects".

and will never be permitted to become human–animal hybrid or chimeric creatures. If, on the other hand, we are talking about the creation of fully formed mature hybrid creatures, then such a situation is clearly more dramatic and may involve different moral issues.[17] However, here also we may be letting our expectations of what humanimal creatures would look like, and hence might be like, be conditioned by mythology, by what we might call the "mermaid myth", which involves the belief that if you mix the genes of a man and a fish you will necessarily make a creature with the recognizable features of both the progenitor creatures—you will make a mermaid, a creature which is half fish and half human.

3.3 How Do We Identify Tissue or Genes as "Animal" or "Human"?

From diet to vaccines, from drugs to xenotransplantation in its various forms, as Giuseppe Testa[18] has noted: "humans and animals have always been exchanging bits of their biological matter, intentionally or by chance, naturally or through artificial aids of various sorts".[19] It is worth remembering that the majority of these encounters do not elicit particular fear or opposition. Diet is a good example: except for vegetarians for whom objections are usually rooted in moral issues concerning animal welfare rather than species mixing, there does not seem to be any preoccupation with the entry of animal genes, cells, tissue, muscle, and other bodily products into our daily metabolism.[20] However, we know, and we learn more almost on a daily basis, that diet influences our body at both genetic and epigenetic levels. "The effect of certain classes of nutrients on the methylation level of our DNA (one of the most meaningful types of epigenetic modification) is just the best defined

---

[17] I use here words also used in *Inter-Species Embryos*.

[18] In this section I have, with his permission, borrowed extensively from the work of my friend and colleague Giuseppe Testa. We have worked together on the ethics of humanimals, but this section on context belongs to Giuseppe. I do not quote him verbatim since I draw these sections from work we wrote together.

[19] Insoo Hyun, Patrick Taylor, Giuseppe Testa, et al., "Ethical Standards for Human-to-Animal Chimera Experiments in Stem Cell Research", *Cell Stem Cell*, vol. 1, no. 2 (16 August 2007): 159–63, at p. 159.

[20] It is true that humans are less sanguine about being eaten by other organic creatures than they are about eating them, but either way we end up with humanimals.

example of the enduring effect of diet on our genetic networks, an effect that might even be passed on to future generations."[21] In fact, if one were consistent in maximizing the purity of human matter, the only dietary choice would be cannibalism.

Vaccines and the various kinds of xenotransplantation are other, more visible, instances of animal–human mixing. Although whole organ xenotransplantations are still in very early experimental phases, porcine neural stem cells have been transplanted into a few patients, and millions of patients worldwide live with heart valves harvested from pigs or cows. In such cases, objections have tended to concentrate on specific dangers (for example the risk of transmitting animal viruses to the human population) rather than on a more general condemnation of human–animal mixing.

A typology of different sorts of human–animal mixing that has some utility is the following:

1. the daily crossing of species boundaries through diet, largely unnoticed and completely normalized in our culture;
2. the widespread use of animal products of various kinds as medical remedies, usually well accepted though with specific safety concerns, as in the various kinds of xenotransplantation;
3. the mixing of human and animal genes as proposed, albeit at a very limited level, in research. And finally
4. the possibility of fully fledged hybrid or chimerical creatures mixing human and animal elements.

The difference is then at the level of the 'fundamental units' that get mixed in the four modalities: animal cells broken down to simple metabolites through the diet; cells that become parts of host tissues through xenotransplantation; and genes that mix up within the host cell in research or in the creation of humanimal creatures.

But is the sharp distinction between these different types of chimeras— and the equally sharp distinction in their moral evaluation—scientifically or ethically justified? The mixing of species is surely better understood as a continuum in which as Testa notes "the lines to be drawn between the acceptable and the non-acceptable do not align neatly with pre-existing

---

[21] Hyun, Taylor, Testa, et al., "Ethical Standards", p. 159.

biological categories (such as genes, cells, or metabolites) and the often inaccurate understandings that underlie them".[22]

We need to reframe the notion of animal or human genes starting from the very problem of defining what it means to say that something is an animal or a human gene. For in the light of the evolutionary conservation of many signalling pathways, 'human' or 'animal' gene can refer only to the fact that these sequences are sourced from a human or an animal.[23] But from this it does not follow that an animal gene, once put into a human, behaves as an independent unit of 'animal agency' or vice versa. And a clear reminder of this point comes from some of the most spectacular results of molecular biology in the 1990s.

In research in the mid-1990s, scientists defined the genetic hierarchy underlying the development of the eye. The experiment was spectacular:

a single gene, transplanted in tissues of the fly embryo such as the wings and the legs, was able to direct the formation of a whole eye, an ectopic eye. And yet, when the human homolog gene was transferred into a mouse to check for its ability to repair the *small eye* mutation, the result remained compelling: again, an eye was formed, testifying to the remarkable evolutionary conservation of genes and developmental pathways.[24]

However, the eye formed from a human gene, when inserted into the mouse 'forms' a mouse eye. Context, in other words, is just as essential as genes.[25] This shows that genes which had their origin in one species may when inserted in another species express themselves in ways adapted to their context. When we mix the genes of different species we do not necessarily mix the characteristics of those species.

Mythology has not prepared us well for the advent of humanimals. Adding fish genes to human embryos is unlikely to give us mermaids, creatures with a woman's upper body and the tail of a fish; adding human genes to horse embryos will probably not create centaurs.

---

[22] Hyun, Taylor, Testa, et al., "Ethical Standards", p. 159.

[23] Hyun, Taylor, Testa, et al., "Ethical Standards", p. 160.

[24] Hyun, Taylor, Testa, et al., "Ethical Standards", p. 160.

[25] G. Halder, P. Callaerts, and W. J. Gehring, "Induction of Ectopic Eyes by Targeted Expression of the Eyeless Gene in Drosophila", *Science*, vol. 267, no. 5205 (1995): 1788–92; G. Oliver and P. Gruss, "Current Views of Eye Development", *Trends in Neuroscience*, vol. 20, no. 9 (1997): 415–21; R. Quiring, U. Walldorf, U. Kloter, and W. J. Gehring, "Homology of the Eyeless Gene of Drosophila to the Small Eye Gene in Mice and Anividia in Humans", *Science*, vol. 265, no. 5173 (1994): 785–9.

Is it too fanciful to suggest that it is the rooted and unreflective priority given to our species in, among other things, our conceptions of human rights and human dignity that are part of the problem here?

3.4 Humans are Already Humanimals

We know we are descended from apes, but we perhaps need to remind ourselves that this descent is seamless and means that our genetic constitution contains a mixture of the genes of all the creatures, all the other species, that are part of the origin of our own transient and probably transitional species.

In his essay "Gaps in the Mind"[26] Richard Dawkins asks us to imagine a contemporary woman. holding her mother's hand on the coast of Africa. She holds her mother's hand, her mother holds *her* mother's, and so on. Each daughter is as much like her mother as daughters usually are. Each person takes up a about a metre, a yard, of space as they hold hands back into the past. In just 300 miles (a small distance into Africa) the imaginary human chain reaches our common ape ancestor. We then need to imagine our ape ancestor holding by her other hand her other daughter and she hers and so on back to the coast. Again each daughter looks as much like her mother as mothers and daughters usually do. By the time the chain reaches back to the coast two contemporary females are looking at one another each holding the hand of her mother stretching in seamless connection back to a common ape ancestor. The two, women shall we call them, looking into each other's eyes are a modern human and a modern chimpanzee.

Dawkins's story reminds us of our ape ancestry and most importantly of the seamless transition between apes and humans. We need to bear in mind another lesson from evolution related to Dawkins's parable and outlined in his essay. That lesson is that it is an accident of evolution that ape species with whom (which?) we humans might have been able, successfully, to breed have not survived. So while the chimpanzee

---

[26] In Richard Dawkins, *The Devil's Chaplain* (London: Phoenix, 2004), pp. 23–31. I use the summary of Dawkins that appears in my *Enhancing Evolution*. I apologize for my frequent recourse to this wonderful example.

who shares a common ancestor with humans probably cannot breed with human beings (at least without technological assistance), there were certainly once non-human apes that, had they survived, could have been procreational partners for us, using "normal" sexual reproduction. To this extent our ability to define ourselves as a species distinct from the other great apes is, in one of the most commonly used definitions of a species, namely, that its members are able to breed successfully with one another but not with other types of animals, an accident of history not an immutable law.

The lesson of Dawkins's example most significant for our present discussion is that *we humans* are humanimals. We are creatures that are as we are because we result from a process—evolution—that has allowed us to evolve from our ape ancestors, not least by incorporating their genes and epigenetic features into our human constitution. In that we incorporate and retain these genes of animal origin, we are indeed also humanimals, a species of interspecies creatures that many call "humans" but which are, whatever else they are, also humanimals. While there may be no obvious point in Dawkins's chain where the mother was an ape and the daughter a human, some mothers (all mothers?) were apes whose daughters or grandchildren were more human than they were or she was. For those who believe that humans are uniquely ensouled, some ape mother without a soul must have given birth to some daughter with a soul (unless souls also admit of degrees). For those who, like Francis Fukuyama, define "what it is to be human" in terms of a factor—Factor X—that humans possess and non-humans do not, there must have been a daughter with Factor X that her mother or great grandmother lacked.[27] But in all of these cases mothers and daughters must have been made of both human and animal elements (at least in the ways that those who object to the creation of humanimals find objectionable).

We should remember that Darwinian evolution is a random and purposeless process which over millions of years effects changes which benefit reproduction but not necessarily anything else—certainly not "fitness for purpose" defined in terms other than those which promote successful propagation of genes.

---

[27] See Francis Fukuyama, *Our Posthuman Future* (London: Profile Books, 2002), p. 160.

3.5 Brave New Worlds

In Shakespeare's *The Tempest*, Miranda, brought up in the company of her father Prospero (a magician) and assorted magical beings, sees ordinary men for the first time and likes what she sees:

> O wonder!
> How many goodly creatures are there here!
> How beauteous mankind is, O brave new world
> that has such people in't.[28]

Since Aldous Huxley brave new worlds have had a bad press, but Miranda is a better guide to the ethics of innovation than Aldous.

Miranda can be seen as celebrating the discovery of her own kind, a celebration of humanity, but I think she sees a deeper truth. The only "men" she has encountered hitherto (besides her father) are the magical intangible Ariel and the loathsome and pitiable Caliban—not much of a choice for a spirited young woman. When she encounters young, good looking, Italian men she is not so much confirming a species preference but demonstrating openness to a better world than the one she currently inhabits, a brave new world. Miranda's quotidian world is magical, and she chooses a better, less familiar world.

The prestige and power of science has sometimes been attributed to the fact that science is just "magic . . . that works!"[29] Insofar as it is, the future as well as the past, is and we may hope will continue to be nothing short of magical and it will have all sorts of unprecedented and we may hope "goodly" creatures in't.

There are already, and in the future there will increasingly be, all kinds of new creatures out there and it will be our business to ensure that they are all as "goodly" as they can be; some will be man-made (rather than man and woman made) resulting from something more akin to construction than sexual reproduction. They may result from synthetic gametes or so-called "synthetic biology", but however synthetic their creation they will be real in every important sense.

---

[28] William Shakespeare, *The Tempest*, Act 5, Scene 1. The Arden Shakespeare, *Complete Works*, ed. Richard Proudfoot, Ann Thomson, and David Scott Kastan (Walton-on-Thames: Thomas Nelson and Sons, 1998).

[29] An epigram that came to me via Frank Cioffi, my undergraduate philosophy tutor in 1966. I don't know where he found it but Internet sources suggest that Kurt Vonnegut may have borrowed it from him or vice versa.

We have already considered humanimals; now we must consider brave new beings which continue the evolutionary process that has resulted in humans. Some will be enhanced humans, but others may be enhanced or at least altered animals. Other creatures will be mixtures, not of human and animal genes or parts, but perhaps humans with technology implanted, (not like the heart pace-makers or prosthetic limbs with which we are familiar but) perhaps with tiny "nanobots" that will dramatically enhance mental powers. Other possibilities include creatures that can literally interface with computers and access data and memory and information processing. Finally increased longevity may eventually result in creatures that are effectively "immortal", an outcome which would certainly constitute a species change since one way of defining humans is as "mortals", creatures that die, as opposed to immortals and Gods which, by hypothesis, do not.[30]

It is just as well that all these new sorts of beings are on the way because in the future it is likely that we will have to face the end of humanity as we know it. We will either have died out altogether, or, we may hope, we will have been replaced by our successors however produced. The end of humanity then is not in itself a concern; making sure that what replaces us is something better is a huge concern.

Since neither our planet nor our sun can endure forever we will have in the long term also to face the necessity of finding a new habitat on another world or indeed of creating such a world.

3.6 Synthetic Biology

One of the most dramatic and important of the new technologies that will eventually produce new creatures is synthetic biology. When people talk about synthetic biology and synthetic life, they may have in mind Frankenstein scientists in the lab making creatures out of old socks and coat hangers, or perhaps some bubbling vat of biochemical "primeval soup" out of which will arise either a monster or a perfect specimen of humanity. The creation of whole complex organisms to rival ourselves is

---

[30] John Harris, "Intimations of Immortality", *Science*, vol. 288, no. 5463 (2000): 59 and John Harris, "Intimations of Immortality: The Ethics and Justice of Life Extending Therapies", in Michael Freeman (ed.), *Current Legal Problems* (Oxford: Oxford University Press, 2002), pp. 65–97.

certainly far in the future! Synthetic biology[31] is the name now often used for a cluster of new technologies in which biomolecular components (natural or synthetic) are newly combined or reorganized in order to create novel genetic and biochemical circuitry, pathways, and ultimately organisms. It may be thought of as a hybrid discipline between science and engineering.

3.7 Made in Our Image

Synthetic biology has caught the imagination not least because it marks the beginnings of what looks like the possibility of manufacturing life forms from scratch and eventually of creating tailor-made creatures in our own image or in principle in the image and with the attributes of anything we like, or at least of anything we can engineer. This is heady stuff, and if it works may eventually give us unprecedented powers, which like all powers may be used for good or evil or simply wasted by lack of use. The storm of interest in synthetic biology has acted as a fascinating counterpoint to the ongoing discussion of the ethics and policy that should govern enhancing technologies of all sorts and human enhancement more generally. Such possibilities have forced us to reconsider who and what we are, and to think more soberly and more objectively about the inevitability of change including what will amount to further evolutionary change and of course change in our understanding of the nature and importance of human rights.

Is either synthetic biology or indeed the disappearance of humanity among the things we should be worried about? How should we begin to address such a question?

3.8 Does Being Human Matter?

Suppose our common ape ancestors in Africa had had the wit and foresight to get together with a simian agenda to block further evolution so that simian nature would have been preserved as "the common

---

[31] In describing synthetic biology I draw on the ideas and research of my colleague John McCarthy, Director of the Manchester Interdisciplinary Biocentre, University of Manchester.

heritage of simian kind".[32] If that had happened we would not be enjoying this pleasant discussion.

What matters then is not being human, but the existence of beings that have those powers and capacities, that have a nature that makes it worthwhile to be alive or to exist.

Whether the new creatures are created by synthetic biology, or by mixing the elements of different species, or indeed through multiple forms of technology, we may, indeed in all probability we must and we will, create new types of creature that might join and we may hope will eventually replace us. Whether or not the non-human persons arise through technology or in the course of further Darwinian evolution, in the future, the far future perhaps, there will be no more humans. We do not need to worry about this so long as we are replaced by something better, by individuals better able to survive, flourish, be curious and inventive, and create a better world and an even better future for those who follow.

3.9 Enhancements and Justice: Synthetic Sunshine

The desire to better ourselves and make ourselves better, is part of the curiosity and need that drives science, one of the oldest and most valuable of the things that characterize persons. An example of an enhancing technology already mentioned in this chapter is synthetic biology, but it is instructive to consider another synthetic product of technology of somewhat more venerable antecedents, synthetic sunshine.

Enhancement technologies,[33] including chemical, genetic, and other high-tech examples, have given and continue to give those who use them or can possess them, an edge, and have often been criticized for the injustice that this supposedly creates. However, before fires, candles, lamps, and other forms of man-made light, most people went to sleep when it got dark. Candles enabled social life and work (unsocial hours)[34]

---

[32] To lightly adapt *The Universal Declaration on the Human Genome and Human Rights*. Published by UNESCO as a pamphlet (3 December 1997) which absurdly endorses "The preservation of the human genome as common heritage of humanity".

[33] For a detailed defence see Harris, *Enhancing Evolution*, on which book I draw in this section. See also Greely et al., "Towards Responsible Use of Cognitive Enhancing Drugs by the Healthy".

[34] It is perhaps another irony that unsocial hours are parasitic upon the concept of social hours, themselves the by-product of the leisure that technology has facilitated.

to continue into and through the night and conferred all sorts of advantages on those able and willing to take advantage to be sure at the expense of those who could or did not take similar advantage.

Contemporary and future enhancements may create problems of injustice both in that they provide a means for some to gain an advantage (those who read by candlelight gain in a way that others do not), and because they may create unfair pressures as a result of the capabilities conferred by enhancement (like the pressure to stay up late and read or work because one can).

The solution is establishing "fair" working hours/working week and provision, at public expense if necessary, of sources of light—not banning the candles! The solution is a combination of regulation and distributive justice, not a Luddite rejection of technology.

Take a different but no less serious example. We, in the United Kingdom, are trying to make kidney transplants available to all who need them, as it is believed the Belgians, the Spanish, and the Austrians have managed to do.[35] Even when that is achieved we know that thousands in the rest of the world cannot obtain the transplants they need. We do not (and surely we should not) say that we will perform no more transplants here until the needs of all those in India can be met. And since we currently do not even have enough kidneys available for our own population, we do not think that fairness demands that we suspend our transplant programme pending a sufficient supply for UK needs.

So when enhancements make life or lives better they are justified if they do just that. If they also confer positional advantage, that is no part of the justification and this fact will always create reasons to distribute such advantages as widely and fairly as possible.

3.10 Human Rights

This brings us back to our starting point with the relevance of humanity to human rights. As this essay on the nature of our humanity has, I hope, indicated, our humanity is both highly contingent and highly problematic. What the idea of human rights does, apart from some rather

---

[35] Statistics from *Eurotransplant* seem to suggest that waiting lists *do* still exist in Belgium and Austria (Eurotransplant does not extend to Spain), although they may be greatly reduced.

problematic self-congratulation for our particular stage of evolution and what we have done with it, is outline a set of entitlements for beings of a particular sort. These entitlements set limits, as Raz has argued, to the powers of the state, but they also set limits as to what individuals may do to one another. Perhaps even more significant they seem to set limits to our capacity for the moral understanding of non-human creatures.

The particular sorts of beings who have this species of important right which we currently call a "human right" are defined, or rather identified, in terms not of species membership or evolutionary stage, but in terms of a particularly interesting set of powers and capacities, certainly possessed by most humans at certain stages of their lives (species typically possessed as it is sometimes said) but also possessed or at least possessable by other creatures. These characteristics I have defined and elaborated elsewhere.[36] They can be seen as emblematic of the scientific endeavour, as characterized by relentless curiosity and the desire to find answers to questions that puzzle us; I prefer to see them in terms of a rather more abstract capacity to value existence. These capacities may well be unique in the universe and are for all we know unique to this planet. If creatures who can value themselves and can value others and can in turn claim respect are to continue, it may be vital both in the short and medium term for those creatures to further evolve or develop by processes other than those of Darwinian or enhancement evolution. This may prove an essential pre-condition to an ability the better to solve the problems that face us and will face our, hopefully improved, successors. And in the long term we may hope that those successors are the sorts of creatures capable of finding other habitats elsewhere in the universe if self-conscious intelligent life of any sort is to continue.

To this end, fetishizing humanity or humanness may be far from conducive to our interests as humans insofar as these extend to the existence and survival of our successors and the continuity of the development of intelligent, sentient creatures.

The most urgent and worrying ethical problems surrounding the uses of new technology, including synthetic biology, are not the dangers of pursuing such research and the innovation that may result. Such dangers attend all research and innovation of whatever nature and must always

---

[36] See Harris, *The Value of Life* and John Harris, "The Concept of the Person and the Value of Life", *Kennedy Institute of Ethics Journal*, vol. 9, no. 4 (1999): 293–308.

be resolved (if they are resolvable) by the best estimation of risk as against benefit. The dangers that have been consistently under-estimated are the dangers of not pursuing such research because a host of feeble and often incoherent objections and objectors have placed themselves in the path of progress towards a better future for humanity and have been given unjustified respect. Turning our back on these possibilities perhaps because, in T. S. Eliot's words,[37] we do not dare "disturb the universe" must not be an option. However, if we do have the courage and the good sense to disturb the universe, at least to the extent of trying to improve on the potentially disastrous vulnerabilities with which Darwinian evolution has left us, then we may indeed live to "hear the mermaids singing, each to each". Perhaps they may even sing to us or to our more fortunate successors.

---

[37] T. S. Eliot, "The Love Song of J. Alfred Prufrock", in T. S. Eliot, *Collected Poems* (London: Faber and Faber, 1963).

4

Moral Enhancement and Freedom

4.1 The Argument

God had important things to say on the subject of moral enhancement.[1] If God's feelings on the subject have been reliably reported by John Milton, the verbatim account to be found in *Paradise Lost*[2] is important because it contains, in a most concise form, many of the most cogent reasons for suspicion as to the viability of moral enhancement as a coherent project, at least as it is being understood in the emerging literature.

Another good reason to listen to[3] Milton's God is his insistence on the necessity and the obligation that we all have to take responsibility for ourselves and for our world, in contradiction of so many recent writers who claim the hubris of attempting to do so exposes us to a myriad of dangers.[4] Equally the failure to exercise such responsibility is far from the path of safety[5] and hot baths.[6]

---

[1] Earlier versions of this chapter appear in John Harris, "Moral Enhancement and Freedom", *Bioethics*, vol. 25, no. 2 (2011): 102–11. I wish to acknowledge the stimulus and support of the iSEI *Wellcome Strategic Programme in the Human Body: its Scope, Limits and Future*. I thank John Coggon for reading earlier drafts and making many valuable suggestions and to Sarah Chan for some incisive suggestions. Thanks are also due to Saira Mian for helpful assistance and insights.

[2] John Milton, *Paradise Lost*, ed. John Leonard (London: Penguin Books, 2000). Milton first published *Paradise Lost* in 1667.

[3] Listen to, yes! Worship or "believe in"—certainly not!

[4] See Francis Fukuyama, *Our Posthuman Future* (London: Profile Books, 2002) and Jürgen Habermas, *The Future of Human Nature* (Cambridge: Polity Press, 2003). It is unusual for me to find God on my side so I am grateful to Milton for listening so intently.

[5] John Harris, *Enhancing Evolution* (Princeton and Oxford: Princeton University Press, 2007).

[6] For the significance of hot baths see Simone Weil, "The *Iliad*, a Poem of Force", in Peter Meyer (ed.), *The Pacifist Conscience* (Harmondsworth: Penguin Books, 1966).

The recent history of bioethics is marked by its commitment; by a move from ethics as etiquette to ethics as engagement.[7] This is all the more vital because from many sources we are receiving warnings of the necessity for early and decisive action to save both humanity and indeed the planet. Climate change, new diseases such as Avian and Swine Flu, the various forms of Creutzfeldt-Jakob Disease (CJD) and HIV/AIDS, Ebola, the population explosion, and increasingly diffused access to weapons of mass destruction all urgently require solutions and are all posing extraordinarily difficult problems and presenting unprecedented dangers. While bioethics is hardly plausible as the saviour science for all these ills, it does have, and has exercised, a vital role in both high-lighting problems and in clearing away many of the tenacious and bad arguments that are constantly produced for avoiding or postponing radical solutions.

Against this background, Moral Enhancement appears as a knight in shining armour equipped to take up arms against a sea of troubles, posed by malevolence and stupidity, and by opposing end them[8] with a molecule of pro-sociality.

In what follows I hope to show why the idea of moral enhancement is being fundamentally misunderstood by many of those interested in further research in this field, and in particular, why mistakes about the nature of both the opportunities it offers and the very nature of "right conduct" are presenting dangers for the present and the future of humanity.

But let's return (or turn) to God for a moment. Famously, in Book III of *Paradise Lost* Milton reports God saying to his "Only begotten Son" that if man is perverted by the "false guile" of Satan he has only himself to blame:

> whose fault?
> Whose but his own? Ingrate, he had of me
> All he could have; I made him just and right,
> Sufficient to have stood, though free to fall.[9]

---

[7] See for example John Harris (ed.), *Bioethics*. Oxford Readings in Philosophy (Oxford and New York: Oxford University Press, 2001), especially the Introduction.

[8] Apologies to William Shakespeare, *Hamlet*, Act III, Scene 1. The Arden Shakespeare, *Complete Works*, ed. Richard Proudfoot, Ann Thomson, and David Scott Kastan (Walton-on-Thames: Thomas Nelson and Sons, 1998), p. 309, lines 57ff.

[9] Milton, *Paradise Lost*, lines 96ff.

These lines have inspired many writers about the human condition and about the precious nature of freedom and in particular of free will. William Golding echoed these famous lines and discussed their theme in his novel *Free Fall*.[10] I first read *Free Fall* as an undergraduate in the 1960s[11] (and it was Golding that pointed me to Milton). Golding asks two crucial questions in that book: "when did I lose my freedom?", and "how did I lose my freedom?" Here is how they are posed on the first page of *Free Fall*:

When did I lose my freedom? For once, I was free. I had power to choose. The mechanics of cause and effect is statistical probability yet surely sometimes we operate below or beyond that threshold. Free will cannot be debated but only experienced, like a colour or the taste of potatoes. I remember one such experience. I was very small and I was sitting on the stone surround of the pool and fountain in the centre of the park. There was bright sunlight, banks of red and blue flowers, green lawn. There was no guilt but only the plash and splatter of the fountain at the centre . . . . The gravelled paths of the park radiated from me: all at once I was overcome by a new knowledge. I could take whichever I would of these paths. There was nothing to draw me down one more than the other. I danced down one for joy in the taste of potatoes. I was free. I had chosen.[12]

Leaving aside Golding's rather suspect views about statistical probability and the assertion that free will cannot be debated (which is demonstrably contradicted in the passage just quoted), Golding vividly illustrates a feeling that surely everyone has had, the feeling of what it is like to be free in an existential sense.[13] With the exhilaration of that feeling, I hope, coursing through our veins (and not, I hope, clouding our judgement) let's return to Milton.

When God says of man that "he had of me all he could have" he qualifies this in two ways. Firstly by the vainglorious claim "I made him just and right", and second by a wonderful analysis of freedom: "sufficient to have stood, though free to fall". Milton's God was certainly overestimating her role in making humankind just, right, and all the

---

[10]   William Golding, *Free Fall* (London: Faber and Faber, 1959).

[11]   While a graduate student in Oxford I had the good fortune to get to know Bill Golding through my friendship with his daughter Judy and with Terrel Carver (later to become Bill's son-in-law) and had the privilege of discussing freedom and many other issues with Golding on a number of occasions.

[12]   Golding, *Free Fall*, p. 5.

[13]   Not "freedom from" but "freedom to". See Isaiah Berlin, "Two Concepts of Liberty", in Isaiah Berlin, *Four Essays on Liberty* (Oxford: Oxford University Press, 1969).

rest, but nature, or more particularly, evolution, has done most of this for us. We have certainly evolved to have a vigorous sense of justice and right, that is, with a virtuous sense of morality. God was, of course, speaking of the fall from Grace, when congratulating herself on making man "sufficient to have stood though free to fall"; she was underlining the sort of existential freedom Golding spoke of which allows us the exhilaration and joy of choosing (and changing at will) our own path through life. And while we are free to allow others to do this for us and to be tempted and to fall, or be bullied, persuaded, or cajoled into falling, we have the wherewithal to stand if we choose. So that when Milton has God say mankind "had of me all he could have", he is pointing out that while his God could have made falling impossible for us, even God could not have done so and left us free. Autonomy surely requires not only the possibility of falling but the freedom to choose to fall, and that same autonomy gives us self-sufficiency; "sufficient to have stood though free to fall".

It would be tempting to conclude at this point that we humans, although we need many forms of enhancement and often desire much more enhancement than we need, do not need and are irrational to seek, specifically *moral* enhancement. This is because we already have not only an extensive moral endowment but because the ways being canvassed to enhance that endowment are unlikely to leave us sufficient to stand though free to fall. However, that would not be quite right either. There are many very attractive and effective forms of moral development including enhancement, available; it is simply that they are not the ones so far being spoken of[14] as either relevant to moral or to neuro-enhancement.

These tried and tested methods include the traditional ones of bringing children up to know the difference between right and wrong, to avoid inflicting pain or suffering on or doing harm to, others, and methods of instilling in them habits of respect for others. These modes of respect include altruism, sensitivity, and consideration and perhaps above all of being able to put ourselves in others' shoes so that we not only understand, but imaginatively experience, what it might be like to be on the receiving end of the conduct of others. Equally, more general education,

---

[14] For example in two essays typical of, indeed exemplary of, recent work on moral enhancement, see notes 17 and 19.

including self-education, wide reading, and engagement with the world and with ways in which the world is mediated (including mass media, computers, and the Internet), are powerful tools of moral development and improvement or enhancement. These must include, of course, sophisticated understanding of cause and effect, in particular of the ways in which to allow things to occur is as effective a way of determining the state of the world as is making positive interventions.[15]

4.1.1 Moral enhancement

In considering moral enhancement, first questions[16] to ask are: what is moral enhancement and what does it have to do with ethical knowledge, if there is such a thing, or with ethical expertise; and what do all of these have to do with knowledge of ethics or morality?

One thing we can say with confidence is that ethical expertise is not "being better at being good", rather it is being better at knowing the good and understanding what is likely to conduce to the good. The space between knowing the good and doing the good is a region entirely inhabited by freedom. Knowledge of the good is sufficiency to have stood, but freedom to fall, is all. Without the freedom to fall, good cannot be a choice and freedom disappears and along with it virtue. There is no virtue in doing what you must.

Those with the insight, sympathy, empathy, understanding, and knowledge to have formed clear ideas of what might conduce to the good are not necessarily better at doing good in any of the ways in which this is possible, including of course making the world a better place. There are many reasons for this and we have space now for only a few.

Some of these are to do with a problem, understood at least since classical Greece, the problem of "akrasia" or weakness of will, one form of which was brilliantly summarized by George Bernard Shaw, when he defined virtue as "insufficient temptation". We know how lamentably bad we are at doing what we know we should. But equally problematic is the fact that this is not, or not wholly, due to lack of moral fibre or resolution, or firmness of purpose. Rather, and again only very partially,

---

[15] See John Harris, *Violence and Responsibility* (London: Routledge & Kegan Paul, 1980).

[16] In this section on moral enhancement I am influenced by the fact that I have just finished discussing them in a new introduction to the paperback edition of my book *Enhancing Evolution*.

it is because we have many purposes, many things to do and experience, and many priorities, of which being good we hope is a part because we hope we do all of these things in a good, a moral way. But of course because we are doing these other things, hopefully with benevolence and good will and good intentions, it is the other purposes for which we also do them that are often, if not more important, at least more at the centre of our attention.

A very fundamental problem, which has not been much discussed in the literature on moral enhancement, is that the sorts of traits or dispositions that seem to lead to wickedness or immorality are also the very same ones required not only for virtue but for any sort of moral life at all.

Tom Douglas, who has a good claim to be one of the "grandfathers" of moral enhancement, has defined the most promising form of this field as "an enhancement that will expectably leave the enhanced person with morally better motives than she had previously".[17] Noting substantial difficulties in identifying "good motives" let alone thinking about how, other than through early education and imaginative engagement with others, or thinking about how to manipulate or improve them, Douglas adopts the interesting expedient of trying to identify what he calls "counter-moral emotions". He identifies at least two: "a strong aversion to certain racial groups" and "the impulse towards violent aggression". Douglas commits himself to the belief that "there are some emotions such that a reduction in the degree to which an agent experiences those emotions would, under some circumstances, constitute a moral enhancement".[18]

There are two substantial problems with this, albeit highly creative, approach. The first is that it seems unlikely that, for example, an aversion to certain racial groups, or to one or more gender or sexual orientation is simply a "brute" reaction, a sort of visceral response, as perhaps is an aversion to spiders. Rather it is likely to be based on false beliefs about those racial or sexual groups and or an inability to see why it might be a problem to generalize recklessly from particular cases. In short, prejudice, as well as rationality, usually has cognitive content and often makes factual claims. Beliefs with cognitive content are for example beliefs that

---

[17] Thomas Douglas, "Moral Enhancement", *Journal of Applied Philosophy*, vol. 25, no. 3 (2008): 228–45. See also: <http://www.ncbi.nlm.nih.gov/pubmed/19132548>.

[18] Douglas, "Moral Enhancement", p. 231.

X is true or Y is false, that A is a danger and B is not, that C is good and D is evil, they are explained by the people that have them in terms of beliefs and ideas, including beliefs about facts which may be, and therefore can often be shown to be, true or false.

The most obvious countermeasure to false beliefs and prejudices is a combination of rationality and education, possibly assisted by various other forms of cognitive enhancement, in addition to courses or sources of education and logic.

Reasons have been advanced for denying or at least circumventing the cognitive elements of certain "immoral beliefs". Ingmar Persson and Julian Savulescu[19] refer to research which reports that "people encode the race of each individual they encounter, and do so via computational processes that appear to be both automatic and mandatory. Encoding by race is a by-product of cognitive machinery that evolved to detect coalitional alliances."[20] While this may be true and while this encoding might be susceptible to disruption, there are some problems with seeing this as a key to moral enhancement. Racism still remains widespread, but is almost everywhere deplored, and in many countries is also against the law. And of course it is racist behaviour, not racist beliefs that are the problem, or the main problem.[21] The most important thing about the prejudices that most, perhaps all of us, have in one form or another, is to recognize them and learn to be ashamed of them and above all not to act on them. The neutralization of the worst effects of racist beliefs is thus probably enhanced by cognitive enhancement. Moreover, it seems likely that racism affects, in a virulent form, only a minority of the world's population and yet all of us have the encoding, so one might think that the encoding cannot be that powerful. Racism has been further reduced dramatically in the last hundred years by forms of moral enhancement including education, public disapproval, knowledge acquisition, and legislation. We thus have a very effective blueprint for the sorts of ways in which we can reduce and hopefully eventually effectively eradicate racism. The blueprint provides a good measure of the effectiveness of

---

[19] Ingmar Persson and Julian Savulescu, "The Perils of Cognitive Enhancement and the Urgent Imperative to Enhance the Moral Character of Humanity", *Journal of Applied Philosophy*, vol. 25, no. 3 (2008): 162–77.

[20] Persson and Savulescu, "The Perils of Cognitive Enhancement", p. 168.

[21] I am grateful to Sarah Chan for reminding me of this important point.

these means and good reason to believe that racism can be defeated by such means without resorting to biological or genetic measures which might have unwanted effects. In the present case such an unwanted effect might be to weaken kinship ties more generally or ones that are unconnected with race for reasons similar to those we are about to discuss.

Moreover, Persson and Savulescu suggest that having:

Suggested that the core moral dispositions . . . have a biological basis and, thus, in principle should be within the reach of biomedical and genetic treatment, the next question is to what extent such treatment is possible in practice. To this question the answer seems to be: only to a very small extent.[22]

To return to Douglas, the second problem with his account is that we would need to be pretty sure that "the reduction in the degree to which the emotion was experienced" could be precisely targeted only on strong aversions to things it is bad to have strong aversions to and not things to which strong aversions are constitutive of sound morality. This problem was effectively articulated by Peter Strawson in a famous essay entitled "Freedom and Resentment".[23] Strawson was not of course concerned with moral enhancement, but rather with the problem of free will. And in the course of combating some absurd forms of determinism, he points out that certain strong emotions, including aversions, are an essential and even desirable part of valuable emotions, motives, or attitudes to others. Could we in short have the sorts of feelings that are appropriate and indeed, it might be argued, necessary to morality, if we did not feel a strong aversion for example, to someone who deliberately and unjustifiably killed or tortured those we love?

While Douglas is right when he claims "there are some emotions such that a reduction in the degree to which an agent experiences those emotions would, under some circumstances, constitute a moral enhancement"[24] this is a very modest claim indeed, and I for one am sceptical that we would ever have available an intervention capable of targeting aversions to the wicked rather than the good. Of course if ever we do have the prospect of such precise and unequivocally good-producing interventions, I will welcome them. But I remain doubtful and remain

---

[22] Persson and Savulescu, "The Perils of Cognitive Enhancement", p. 172.

[23] Peter Strawson, "Freedom and Resentment", *Proceedings of the British Academy*, vol. 48 (1960): 187–211.

[24] Douglas, "Moral Enhancement", p. 231.

worried about the prospect of weakening, possibly essential and essentially moral, responses. This is a "baby and bathwater" problem which may prove soluble; I hope it will, but fear it may be intractable.

As we have seen, there are substantial issues of liberty which would also need to be resolved and which could conceivably be threatened by any measures that make the freedom to do immoral things impossible, rather than simply making the doing of them wrong and giving us moral, legal, and prudential reasons to refrain.

4.2 The Analysis

4.2.1 Purity and danger

Ingmar Persson and Julian Savulescu have produced a characteristically bold and simultaneously an intriguing and a worrying manifesto for the urgency and importance of moral enhancement. In a paper whose title sums up the agenda,[25] they are pessimistic, to the point of paranoia,[26] about the merits of cognitive enhancement and seem to argue that efforts to improve cognitive powers and capacities should be put on hold until moral enhancement is perfected and infallible and made not only universally available, but comprehensively mandatory. One problem with such an approach is that there are good reasons (which we have reviewed and will return to in due course) to believe moral enhancement must, in large part, consist of cognitive enhancement.

Persson and Savulescu summarize their argument in five main claims:

1. It is comparatively easy to cause great harm, much easier than to benefit to the same extent.
2. With the progress of science, which would be speeded up by cognitive enhancement it becomes increasingly possible for small groups of people, or even single individuals, to cause great harms to millions of people, e.g. by means of nuclear or biological weapons of mass destruction.

---

[25] Persson and Savulescu, "The Perils of Cognitive Enhancement".

[26] Elizabeth Fenton has also criticized Persson and Savulescu's arguments against cognitive enhancement, although she is more sanguine than I am as to the possible merits and success of genetic or biological cognitive enhancement. See Elizabeth Fenton, "The Perils of Failing to Enhance: A Response to Persson and Savulescu", *Journal of Medical Ethics*, vol. 36, no. 3 (2010): 148–51.

3. Even if only a tiny fraction of humanity is immoral enough to want to cause large scale harm by weapons of mass destruction in their possession, there are bound to be some such people in a huge human population, as on Earth, unless humanity is extensively morally enhanced. (Or the human population is drastically reduced, or there is mass genetic screening and selection, though we take it that there is no morally acceptable way of achieving these sufficiently effectively.)

4. A moral enhancement of the magnitude required to ensure that this will not happen is not sufficiently possible at present and is not likely to be possible in the near future.

5. Therefore, the progress of science is in one respect for the worse by making likelier the misuse of ever more effective weapons of mass destruction, and this badness is increased if scientific progress is speeded up by cognitive enhancement, until effective means of moral enhancement are found and applied.

Persson and Savulescu conclude that:

If safe moral enhancements are ever developed, there are strong reasons to believe that their use should be obligatory... That is, safe, effective moral enhancement would be compulsory.

Now of course the mischief is in the meaning . . . in this case of the words "safe and effective" but before seeing just how much mischief might be possible it is worth taking a moment to examine the plausibility of Persson and Savulescu's five main claims.

4.2.2 First claim

1. It is comparatively easy to cause great harm, much easier than to benefit to the same extent.

This seems superficially true, so that when Persson and Savulescu draw attention to the Virginia Tech killings in 2007 and say:

Seung-Hui Cho killed 32 people in the worst civil shooting in US history. Cho used two semiautomatic handguns. The actual killings took place in a couple of minutes. It is almost never possible to save 32 lives in the same period of time.[27]

we are inclined to accept it at face value.

---

[27] Persson and Savulescu, "The Perils of Cognitive Enhancement", p. 173.

But when we stop nodding at the obvious, but limited, relevance of such an example and examine it, this claim shows itself to be totally implausible. Raising the alarm when a fire is noticed in a school so that the building can be successfully evacuated or overpowering hijackers or terrorists who would destroy a plane in flight, often saves as many and usually more lives in as many minutes. So that when Persson and Savulescu say: "It is almost never possible to save 32 lives in the same period of time" I am sorry to have to say that this is manifestly absurd.

On Saturday, 26 December 2009 Umar Abdul Mutallab tried to set off a bomb on Flight 253 carrying 290 people while it was attempting to land in Detroit. Jasper Schuringa became an international hero for thwarting this attempt and probably saving every life on the plane. This is the report of the incident from *The Observer*, a London newspaper, of the following day:

"When [it] went off, everybody panicked," said Jasper Schuringa, a Dutch film director travelling to the US to visit friends. "Then someone screamed, 'Fire! Fire!' I saw smoke rising from a seat . . . I didn't hesitate. I just jumped." Schuringa said he heard a sound similar to a firework going off and looked across the aisle at the suspect who had a blanket on his lap attempting to ignite an object he was holding. "It was smoking and there were flames coming from beneath his legs," he said. "I searched on his body parts and he had his pants open. He had something strapped to his legs."

Schuringa and the cabin crew then dragged Mutallab, a 23-year-old Nigerian, to the front of the plane, where he was restrained until landing. Mutallab reportedly told intelligence agents who began interrogating him after he was taken to hospital strapped to a stretcher that he had an explosive powder strapped to his leg. He was trying to set off the device with a syringe filled with liquid.[28]

We are obviously not going to quibble over the meaning of the words "same period of time". I am sure Mr Schuringa did not time the event, but the issue is the plausibility of the claim "It is comparatively easy to cause great harm, much easier than to benefit to the same extent". The example of Flight 253[29] shows that nine times the number of people, as in the Persson and Savulescu example, can be saved in a comparable period of time; and this is not an isolated example. The case of the infamous shoe bomber who was overpowered by crew and passengers

---

[28] <http://www.guardian.co.uk/world/2009/dec/27/abdul-muttalab-flight-253-terrorist-al-qaida>, accessed 11 April 2010.

[29] <http://news.bbc.co.uk/1/hi/uk/8431499.stm>, accessed 11 April 2010.

while trying to set off a bomb and which anyone who has had to remove their shoes at airport security will remember with affection,[30] was similar, and there are many more.

More obviously, the voting of huge sums of money for famine relief or aid work following a tsunami or earthquake, or to allocate vaccines (for example the provision of 35 million doses of the Tamiflu vaccine for the UK population against a pandemic)[31] is the work of a few minutes, but might save thousands, even millions of lives. In the event, of course, the influenza pandemic was much milder than feared and most of the antiviral reserves remain for another day. Vaccine programmes, while not instantly implementable, are quick and dramatic ways to save millions of lives. Whatever the death toll of a disaster, once methods of preventing a recurrence are found, the implementation of those methods almost certainly saves as many if not more lives as might have been threatened by the disaster. This is because preventive measures probably forestall not only this year's disaster but next year's and the following years' as well. For if the preventive measures are permanent, as is likely in the case of smallpox and polio for example, then arguably an indefinite time-sensitive multiplication of the death toll relates plausibly and proportionately to the lives saved. Whether or not this is an acceptable basis for a precise calculation, it is surely unlikely that the lives saved will be fewer in number than those previously lost in a permanently prevented pandemic. Thus:

Smallpox continued to ravage Europe, Asia, and Africa for centuries. In Europe, near the end of the eighteenth century, the disease accounted for nearly 400,000 deaths each year, including five kings. Of those surviving, one-third were blinded. The worldwide death toll was staggering and continued well into the twentieth century, where mortality has been estimated at 300 to 500 million. This number vastly exceeds the combined total of deaths in all world wars.[32]

And arguably the initiation of the WHO plan to eradicate smallpox saved at least as great a proportion of the world's population as that estimated to be threatened by it.

---

[30] <http://en.wikipedia.org/wiki/Richard_Reid_(shoe_bomber)>, accessed 11 April 2010.
[31] <http://news.bbc.co.uk/1/hi/health/8606032.stm>, accessed 11 April 2010.
[32] <http://www.infoplease.com/cig/dangerous-diseases-epidemics/smallpox-12000-years-terror.html>, accessed 11 April 2010.

In 1967, when WHO launched an intensified and effective plan to eradicate smallpox, this disease threatened 60 per cent of the world's population, killing every fourth victim, and scarring or blinding most survivors.

As of the last century, as Persson and Savulescu confirm, smallpox is regarded as entirely eradicated. So much for the claim that: "It is comparatively easy to cause great harm, much easier than to benefit to the same extent"! Persson and Savulescu can certainly be forgiven for this error; it is all too easy to accept a dramatic cliché which seems to illustrate something one is tempted to believe, and I have done so many times myself. It is, however, useful to lay this particular "canard" to rest once and for all.

Persson and Savulescu quite rightly make great play with the dangers of biological weapons and the possibilities of bioterrorism.

The polio virus has now been artificially constructed ... More frighteningly scientists have modified mousepox to make it lethal in 100% of mice ... Voltaire estimated that smallpox killed around 20% of the French population in his day. It was eradicated last century from the globe by vaccination ... Genetic engineering of smallpox could create a new strain which would wipe out all or most of humanity.

So it could, and cognitively enhanced science might create a vaccine in time to prevent it. This seems a telling example; but what does it tell? The answer is that it tells rather against the Persson/Savulescu thesis than for it. First it shows that just as a disease like smallpox is an effective killer, vaccines against it are equally successful ways of saving lives. How long did it take to kill 20 per cent of the French population in Voltaire's day? How long did it take to save those same numbers with a vaccine? These are complex questions and because of ambiguities about when a lethal agent operates and when a protective measure actually does the protecting, they are probably not even answerable questions.

But if we compare the time taken by Seung-Hui Cho to kill thirty-two people and the time it would take to administer say thirty-two doses of polio vaccine via sugar lump to a queue of children, the time difference would not be significant. Add to this the numbers killed by polio and the numbers vaccinated we can see that it is often comparatively easy and not time consuming to save great numbers of lives.

Of course it might be claimed that the development of effective vaccines, for example against polio and smallpox, took a great deal of time, but so did the development of semi-automatic handguns. From the first use of firearms somewhere between China in the ninth century and medieval Europe in the thirteenth century to today is a very long time indeed. The fact that once developed, both vaccines and semi-automatic firearms, are fast acting emphasizes the similarities rather than the differences.

What seems clear is that the time the killing or the saving takes is trivial compared with the effectiveness of each. No generalizations to the effect that damage is always or even often quicker than repair, or prevention slower in taking effect than what it prevents, are helpful in addressing the potency of dangers or the probability of defences against them being effective. We can be confident in our conclusion that claim one is false; not least because it depends on upholding a version of the acts/omissions distinction which I am sure that Savulescu at least, rejects. For if a mad or bad individual can destroy the world instantly by setting off a doomsday machine, then a good consequentialist can save the world as quickly by killing him (or morally enhancing him) the moment before he can do so or at any time before that! And this sort of prevention is a recurrent theme of Savulescu's work.

4.2.3 Claims 2 and 3 need to be considered together

> 2. With the progress of science, which would be speeded up by cognitive enhancement it becomes increasingly possible for small groups of people, or even single individuals, to cause great harms to millions of people, e.g. by means of nuclear or biological weapons of mass destruction.
>
> 3. Even if only a tiny fraction of humanity is immoral enough to want to cause large scale harm by weapons of mass destruction in their possession, there are bound to be some such people in a huge human population, as on Earth, unless humanity is extensively morally enhanced . . .

Essentially this is the claim that it only takes one bad man to spoil things for the rest of us. This may well be true, in the sense that its possibility cannot be ruled out, but it is not just the wicked that present problems of this sort. Moreover, it is not clear either that speeding up the progress of science through cognitive enhancement exacerbates the process, nor that moral enhancement has much prospect of eradicating this possibility, indeed the reverse may be true. We need to remember that any tool or technology can be abused or misused and that accidents and negligence can already routinely cause, or threaten, harms on a massive scale (Three Mile Island, Chernobyl).

If, and insofar as, it is true that scientific progress increases the power of individuals to do harm, it is not clear that moral enhancement if and when it might be possible to imagine it to have become "safe" and "effective", will much reduce this danger. Although I am sure that Persson and Savulescu would acknowledge that mad, as well as bad, individuals can cause harm, they talk throughout their paper almost exclusively as if the danger was from wickedness, perhaps because they want to encourage the prioritization of moral enhancement as a field of study.

4.2.4 The village idiot

Now add to this that the danger comes not simply from the malevolent, but from another important category of disastrous individuals. Persson and Savulescu refer to the work of Martin Rees. Now Rees is famous for (among many other things) his elevation of the "village idiot" to global status. In his fascinating book *Our Final Century*[33] Rees catalogues the disasters which might, if the causes of them are not addressed, lead to the end of human life on this planet. Rees considers the role of malevolence or wickedness but also warns of the dangers posed by incompetence or stupidity.

We are entering an era when a single person can, by one clandestine act, cause millions of deaths or render a city uninhabitable for years, and when a malfunction in cyberspace can cause havoc worldwide to a significant segment of the economy: air transport, power generation, or the financial system. Indeed disaster could be caused by someone who is merely incompetent rather than malign.[34]

Rees glossed these remarks at the Hay festival in 2006: "in a global village there will be global village idiots, just one could be too many", and he concluded that there is a real concern about whether our civilization can be safeguarded without us having to sacrifice too much in terms of privacy, diversity, and individualism. I agree with Rees about this, and would add dangers to liberty and autonomy. But I run too far ahead; let's complete our discussion of Persson and Savulescu.

4.2.5 Claims 4 and 5 need to be considered together

> 4. A moral enhancement of the magnitude required to ensure that this will not happen is not sufficiently possible at present and is not likely to be possible in the near future.

---

[33] Martin Rees, *Our Final Century* (London: Arrow Books, 2004).

[34] Rees, *Our Final Century*, p. 61.

> 5. *Therefore, the progress of science is in one respect for the worse by making likelier the misuse of ever more effective weapons of mass destruction, and this badness is increased if scientific progress is speeded up by cognitive enhancement, until effective means of moral enhancement are found and applied.*

These final two claims are interesting. The first, that moral enhancement by new and more radical means than education, knowledge acquisition, and scientific progress is at best a long way off seems right to me; but the alleged sequitur is definitely of the "non" variety. One of the reasons for this is that claim 4 not only notes how far off moral enhancement of any new kind is likely to be, but refers to a "moral enhancement of the magnitude required to ensure that" disaster is avoided. There are many reasons to believe that such "ensurance" and the assurance that follows from it, are impossible, not least because failures in any human intervention are not only possible but are arguably inevitable. There is no such thing as *ensuring* safety.

Even more significant are the costs of delay. While we wait patiently with Persson and Savulescu for the mid to far future perfection of genetic or biological moral enhancement, and while we put on hold the cognitive enhancement that might accelerate scientific advance and the discovery and innovation it produces, "stuff" or even events happen![35] That stuff will be the minute by minute, day by day accumulation of premature death and suffering from causes that cognitive enhancement and the resulting innovation might have prevented.

In my book *Violence and Responsibility*, published over thirty-five years ago now, I was concerned with our responsibility for harms which we might prevent or might have prevented. I insisted that, for example, the violence of political change must be evaluated against what the social historian Barrington Moore Jr called "the violence of normal times". "To dwell on the horrors of revolutionary violence while forgetting that of 'normal' times", he said, is "merely partisan hypocrisy".[36]

---

[35] Donald Rumsfeld was by no means the first to give this memorable truism an epigrammatic validity. The British Prime Minister Harold Macmillan gave this idea slightly more elegant expression in response to a journalist who allegedly asked him what might blow the government off-course? He replied: "events dear boy, events" and much as it goes against the grain they were both right.

[36] W. Barrington Moore Jr., *The Social Origins of Dictatorship and Democracy* (Harmondsworth: Penguin Books, 1969), p. 103.

Barrington Moore Jr warned that the death toll of, for example, the revolutionary terror of the French Revolution, must be seen as a response to "the prevailing social order" which "always grinds out its toll of unnecessary death year after year".[37] We are attuned now to be sensitive to the costs of delay in instituting not only social reform that might prevent unnecessary death and suffering, but the delays that result from failures to turn discovery rapidly into innovation, and to ensure that innovation results in products in the clinic and the marketplace that will save and ameliorate lives. Persson and Savulescu refer to the work of Jonathan Glover, although not in this regard, but they might also have referred to earlier work of Julian Savulescu. It is an irony that Savulescu is here advocating the sort of delays in adopting new technology and medical innovation which certainly will cost lives, delays of the sort that in the past he has been vigilant to oppose.[38] Of course if haste will cost more lives than delay we have good reasons for a precautionary approach. In the present case, as Persson and Savulescu admit, there is not only no immediate prospect of moral enhancement but we have literally no idea how long (if ever) it will take to perfect. On the other hand we have daily evidence of the record of science and technology in preventing and treating disease and premature death and in dramatic increases in life expectancy.

Moreover if Martin Rees is right this cannot be *ensured* because it is unlikely that moral enhancement will affect the proverbial "village idiot", nor the sort of disaster that might result from negligence or miscalculation. Rees's book cites many examples of how much room there is for the disastrous miscalculation of the level of risk inherent in many apparently benign or "morally neutral" technologies. The question then becomes one of whether forgoing the benefits that might accrue from accelerating science via cognitive enhancement (including the rapid development of antidotes to engineered diseases and other bio-weapons and biohazards, better insights into how to combat the worst effects of climate change, and reliable methods of predicting asteroid strikes and developing methods of diverting the asteroids) will prove amenable to a scientific or technological "fix". While we can be sure of none of these things it

---

[37] Barrington Moore Jr., *Social Origins*, p. 103.
[38] See for example Julian Savulescu, "Justice, Fairness and Enhancement", *Annals of the New York Academy of Sciences*, vol. 1093 (2006): 321–38.

would not simply be a brave individual but surely a reckless one who would bet against the overall utility of scientific advance and cognitive enhancement.

Julian Savulescu is one of the smartest people I know. Until this moment I had no reason to think of him as, for this reason, also one of the most dangerous. Should I also begin to look on my most talented students with equal suspicion and do my best to sabotage their cognitive advancement? I hope I have found reasons in this chapter both to continue to admire Julian, and continue to encourage my best students. Indeed as Elizabeth Fenton has pointed out, "it is difficult not to take [Persson's and Savulescu's pessimism] to imply that unless and until we further understand moral enhancement, we should try to slow scientific progress".[39] She might have gone further and pointed out that their extreme risk aversion would justify not only retarding scientific progress but retarding the cognitive powers of people as well.

4.2.6 Milton revisited

Although Persson and Savulescu say: "True, there are also respects in which scientific progress accelerated by cognitive enhancement would be for the better, by protecting us against threats posed by asteroids, epidemics etc. We have not attempted to settle definitely the balance between these good and bad respects" this is disingenuous and is at odds with what they say elsewhere. In talking about the dangers from cognitive enhancement for example they say:

it is enough if very few of us are malevolent or vicious enough to use this power for all of us to run an unacceptable increase of the risk of death and disaster. To eliminate this risk, cognitive enhancement would have to be accompanied by a *moral* enhancement which extends to *all* of us, since such moral enhancement could reduce malevolence.[40]

Here they are explicit that cognitive enhancement "would have to be accompanied by a *moral* enhancement which extends to *all* of us" before the risks of cognitive enhancement would be other than "unacceptable".

Notice also that they talk of the *elimination* of the risk in a context where moral enhancement which *extends to all of us* will only, at best,

---

[39] Fenton, "The Perils of Failing to Enhance", p. 149.
[40] Persson and Savulescu, "The Perils of Cognitive Enhancement", p. 166.

reduce malevolence. So even in the most ideal scenario in their terms, a risk which obtains if only one malevolent person escapes is still, for them, massively significant. So we have a strategy to eliminate a danger which has to be universally applied but only reduces (but not eliminates) the risk of the danger, the risk of which is defined in terms of the people who pose the danger (whose numbers are already admittedly very small)—"it is enough if *very few* of us are malevolent"!

But of course cognitive enhancement is also well calculated to speed up the sorts of advances that can, do, and will save lives. We would have to be very sure of the probability of its negative effects to be justified in ignoring the positive ones.

My own reading of the balance here is rather different. Science, innovation, and knowledge production, particularly education, are I believe our chief hope of finding solutions to the most threatening sources of probable mass destruction and are, moreover, our only proven forms of moral enhancement to date (and have proved very effective). Add to this the point, emphasized by Martin Rees, that evil is not the most probable source of catastrophe, and that threats not amenable to moral enhancement such as asteroids, new diseases, climate change and idiocy, inadvertence and negligence of all sorts, are equally likely, perhaps more likely to produce disaster, and we have a different agenda. This agenda is to reject the idea of putting on hold cognitive enhancement until moral enhancement is in place to rein it in. Rather we must embrace reliable forms of cognitive enhancement in the hope and reasonable expectation that they are our best prospect of self-defence including whatever element of self-defence may eventually result from moral enhancement. Indeed cognitive enhancement might reasonably be expected to reduce idiocy, even of the common or village variety!

Milton reminded us that we have been made with both freedom and a powerful sense of justice and the right, and I am sure that Darwinian evolution rather than God is the force responsible. Either way we have what we need, both to know the good and to try to do the good. This knowledge, like all knowledge, can be improved upon and I believe we should look to improve our capacity for knowledge as effectively and as fast as possible. But the other part of Milton's insight is the crucial role of personal liberty and autonomy: that sufficiency to stand is worthless, literally morally bankrupt, without freedom to fall. Again my own view is that I, like so many others, would not wish to sacrifice freedom for survival. I might of course lack the courage to make that choice when and if the time comes. I hope, however, that I would, and I believe, on grounds that have more eloquently been so often stated by lovers of freedom throughout history, that freedom is certainly as precious, perhaps more precious than life.

Persson and Savulescu end their paper with a truly chilling reference to C. S. Lewis's stories for children and the frightful "Deplorable Word".

This is a 'magical curse which ends all life in the world except that of the one who speaks it' . . . If we all knew the Deplorable Word, the world would likely not last long. The Deplorable Word may arrive soon, in the form of nanotechnology or biotechnology. Perhaps the only solution is to engineer ourselves so that we can never utter it, or never want to utter it.[41]

Ironically and perhaps self-defeatingly it would have to be biotechnology, and possibly cognitively enhanced biotechnology, that would give us the power to engineer ourselves into losing our freedom to innovate in biotechnology in this truly deplorable way. I think we have to hope for something better and perhaps someone better than C. S. Lewis to analyse the dangers.

Persson and Savulescu may well be right, but we will only know that once moral enhancement has been perfected and only if thereafter bad men, madmen, and idiots have ceased to commit or attempt acts of mass destruction. The perfection of moral enhancement is admitted by Persson and Savulescu "not likely to be possible in the near future". I believe it will never be possible to the extent the Persson/Savulescu thesis requires, or indeed that Tom Douglas believes; both for reasons already given and because moral enhancement has little prospect of preventing idiocy—but of course I could be wrong! Even if Persson and Savulescu have made the better bet, we will have to wait a long time to know which of us is right, a long time for non-traditional moral enhancement to be possible and then another, possibly even longer, period of time for it to become universal and then another even longer time than that to have any idea whether or not it is working. Meanwhile wickedness and idiocy not to mention human inadequacy will continue to grind out its daily death toll, a toll that might in all this time have been dramatically reduced by discoveries accelerated by cognitive enhancement. Moreover,

---

[41] Persson and Savulescu, "The Perils of Cognitive Enhancement", p. 175.

these discoveries might save (might have saved) us from a very large class of dangers of mass destruction not attributable to malice, and therefore not susceptible to moral enhancement, such as disease, asteroid strikes, and climate change. I don't believe it would be rational to bet on moral enhancement and against accelerating our ability to deal with . . . literally anything, an ability which is likely to stem, with immediate effect, from cognitive enhancement whether it takes the form of greater alertness or wakefulness in pilots and long-distance drivers and emergency medical staff or better decision-making from workers who have to function in all sorts of demanding situations.[42]

A strategy that leaves us free to search for solutions to problems we cannot as yet even foresee, one that permits us to use techniques of cognitive enhancement to accelerate that process, and one which leaves us free to find, and equipped to implement, those solutions as quickly as possible is a better bet. It is surely better to remain sufficient to stand and to hang on to our precious freedom to fall.

---

[42] Henry Greely, Barbara Sahakian, John Harris, Ron Kessler, Michael Gazzaniga, Philip Campbell, and Martha Farah, "Towards Responsible Use of Cognitive Enhancing Drugs by the Healthy", *Nature*, vol. 456, no. 7223 (2008): 702–5.

5

Taking Liberties with Free Fall

In his "Moral Enhancement, Freedom, and What We (Should) Value in Moral Behavior" David DeGrazia takes issue with a number of arguments that are now to be found in this book. He sets out to defend Moral Bioenhancement (MB) from a number of critics, me prominently among them. He has some important points of critique against my suggestions in the previous chapter that some forms of purported Moral Bioenhancement are inimical to freedom. Here he sets out his stall:

Many scholars doubt what I assert: that there is nothing inherently wrong with MB. Some doubt this on the basis of a conviction that there is something inherently wrong with biomedical enhancement technologies in general. Chief among their objections are the charges that (1) biomedical enhancement is unnatural, (2) use of biomedical enhancements evinces an insufficient appreciation for human "giftedness", and (3) biomedical enhancements pose a threat to personal identity. Elsewhere I have attempted to neutralize these objections. Here I will address a set of concerns that are directed at MB in particular and appeal to the nature and value of human freedom.[1]

Let me make clear at once that I do not believe there is anything inherently wrong with Moral Bioenhancement. I have been an advocate for human enhancement for over thirty years, writing four books defending such enhancements.[2] The most recent of these published in 2007 covers much the same ground as Allen Buchanan's 2011 book cited by DeGrazia.[3] Unlike Buchanan, however, I do not define enhancements in

---

[1] David DeGrazia, "Moral Enhancement, Freedom, and What We (Should) Value in Moral Behaviour", *Journal of Medical Ethics*, vol. 40, no. 6 (2014): 361–8, at p. 361.

[2] John Harris, *The Value of Life* (London: Routledge, 1985); John Harris, *Wonderwoman and Superman: The Ethics of Human Biotechnology* (Oxford: Oxford University Press, 1992); John Harris, *On Cloning* (London: Routledge, 2004); John Harris, *Enhancing Evolution* (Princeton and Oxford: Princeton University Press, 2007).

[3] Allen Buchanan, *Beyond Humanity?* (New York: Oxford University Press, 2011).

terms of the intention or the motivation of those who produce them, but rather in terms of their effect. I must also make clear that like DeGrazia I have also, for a very long time, attempted to neutralize objections 1–3 listed in the passage just cited.[4]

DeGrazia introduces his critique of my approach like this:

I will construe Harris' argument and similar arguments as directed entirely at motivation-based MB—though I will hereafter omit the qualifier, "motivation-based." (Certainly, these arguments do not apply to embryo selection, which cannot alter—and therefore cannot affect the freedom of—particular individuals.)

According to Harris, MB would eliminate the freedom to choose to do wrong—to "fall"—and therefore the freedom to choose rightly. With freedom, he thinks, goes virtue. His position assumes that virtue is intrinsically, not just instrumentally, valuable. Perhaps that is correct.

It is very odd to think of my critique of MB as directed at "motivation-based MB" since I do not believe, and have never suggested, that MB as it currently works and in the form that I have criticized it, operates on anything so sophisticated and complex as "motivation". It operates on, and indeed claims to operate on, "pro-social attitudes" of, I have argued, a monumentally crude sort.[5] Moral enhancement does not make nor even attempt to make better people; it may if it is lucky make people more likely to avoid aggressive behaviour but luck might just as easily go the wrong way as far as morality properly so called, is concerned.

Moreover, the "virtue" of which I speak in the passage quoted, is the virtue of possessing the ability to choose rationally and freely according to principles and practices which are plausible as candidates for moral action. I would not call these "intrinsic goods".

Nor am I claiming that anything, except possibly death and taxes, entirely eliminates freedom. Rather, as DeGrazia rightly interprets me, it "would eliminate some significant measure of our freedom and thereby of virtue—and that this loss would be unacceptable".

---

[4] Harris, *The Value of Life*; Harris, *Wonderwoman and Superman*; Harris, *On Cloning*; Harris, *Enhancing Evolution*.

[5] John Harris, "Moral Enhancement and Freedom", *Bioethics*, vol. 25, no. 2 (2011): 102–11; John Harris, "Moral Progress and Moral Enhancement", *Bioethics*, vol. 27, no. 5 (2013): 285–90; John Harris, "What It's Like to be Good", *Cambridge Quarterly of Healthcare Ethics*, vol. 21, no. 3 (2012): 293–305; John Harris, "'Ethics is for Bad Guys!': Putting the 'Moral' into Moral Enhancement", *Bioethics*, vol. 27, no. 3 (2013): 169–73; Sarah Chan and John Harris, "Moral Enhancement and Pro-Social Behaviour", *Journal of Medical Ethics*, vol. 37, no. 3 (2011): 130–1.

DeGrazia then digresses into a long tutorial on the free will versus determinism debate, which seems to me to be wholly beside the point. All this talk about free will, determinism, and compatibilism is just smoke and mirrors in this context. I make no assumptions about the viability of a non-deterministic account of free will and for what it's worth think some version of compatibilism is probably right. I am talking about common or garden freedom, the freedom which any rational person accepts is inhibited by threats, diminished by the fore-closure of options, and enhanced by education and civil liberties. Indeed my claim is MB acts like a deep-seated irrational prejudice, like racism, sexism, or speciesism. It clouds judgement, making the subject much less able to choose rationally and weigh alternatives from a moral perspec-tive. It may produce moral behaviour, in the sense of behaviour that is *de facto* right or good all things considered, but not behaviour that is informed by moral judgement, which I take to be behaviour best *calcu-lated*, *judged* by a moral agent to have that effect.

DeGrazia claims:

> Moreover, in the case of competent adults deciding to take MB, they choose the means to improved motivation—just as they might choose to go to a consciousness-raising group that applies a certain amount of psychological pressure. Even if some significant causal work is done in either case by something outside of one's agency, one is not a passive subject of this influence but instead actively welcomes it.

I do not of course accept that MB is currently any sort of means to improved motivation although I do not rule out the possibility that more sophisticated methods might be. But, consider that the racist usually actively welcomes his urge to select against blacks or Jews or whomso-ever, in choosing between candidates for a job or public office. My claim is indeed entirely the converse of this. I argue that MB so far from raising consciousness, may well dull it to the point where the individual is no longer choosing at all, at least in any sense in which the word "autono-mous" may be coupled with the word "choice".

When DeGrazia says: "On the compatibilist conception of freedom, acting freely requires not perfect independence from causal influence—which is impossible on this conception—but the right sort of relationship between one's preferences and action as well as the absence of certain sorts of freedom-subverting conditions" this is absolutely right and I have never suggested that there is ever any such thing as "perfect independence from causal influence". What MB seems to do, at least when attempted by the manipulation of levels of serotonin or oxytocin is, I have argued,[6] inhibit the individual from considering which course of action best fulfils their moral preferences and objectives "all things considered". The presence of these molecules in particular doses, is indeed "freedom-subverting"; if it were not, it is unlikely they would have the effects vaunted by their advocates, that is, effects which operate independently of the will or of judgement; unlike education for example which provides the basis for voluntary choices. Here DeGrazia and I may genuinely disagree about the facts.

DeGrazia goes on to defend his own common or garden conception of "free action" like this:

> "A autonomously performs intentional action X if and only if (1) A does X because she prefers to do X, (2) A has this preference because she (at least dispositionally) identifies with and prefers to have it, and (3) this identification has not resulted primarily from influences that A would, on careful reflection, consider alienating."
> I maintain that any action that meets these conditions is genuinely free. Yet there is no reason to suppose that the moral behavior of those who have undergone MB would necessarily or routinely fail these criteria. In the case in which I render assistance where doing so is inconvenient but morally required, I would not consider the influence of MB on my motivation to be alienating. I welcomed this influence.[7]

DeGrazia's definition of free action seems deficient because of the ambiguity and subjectivity of condition 3. Would a racist on careful reflection be likely to be able to see that his prejudice was "alienating", indeed would he even recognize it as prejudice?

When DeGrazia says: "In the case in which I render assistance where doing so is inconvenient but morally required, I would not consider the influence of MB on my motivation to be alienating. I welcomed this influence" he is being somewhat disingenuous. He may well have welcomed the influence but that may be because of the influence of the influence, not because it is the right thing to do all things considered. Does it or doesn't it inhibit the consideration of all things relevant to the

---

[6] Harris, "Moral Enhancement and Freedom"; Harris, "Moral Progress and Moral Enhancement"; Harris, "What It's Like to be Good"; Harris, "'Ethics is for Bad Guys!': Putting the 'Moral' into Moral Enhancement"; Chan and Harris, "Moral Enhancement and Pro-Social Behaviour".

[7] DeGrazia, "Moral Enhancement, Freedom, and What We (Should) Value in Moral Behaviour", p. 366.

choice at hand? My claim is that while the influence is indeed on motivation (if that term is understood, as it sometimes is, simply as a mainspring of action), this "motivation" does not meet standards of moral reasoning for the simple and sufficient reason that it does not meet standards of reasoning at all. The intervention is designed to bypass reasoning and act directly on attitudes. When such attitudes are manipulated, not only is freedom subverted but morality is bypassed. Little wonder that someone in the grip of an attitude-directing molecule would be unlikely to do anything but welcome the fact that they had done what they wanted to do or "felt like" doing. (How apposite our idioms sometimes are!) I, however, want them to be free (free-er) to consider at the time whether this motivation is in fact directing them to the best outcome morally speaking . . . the best outcome "all things considered".

"Ability to act otherwise, or freedom to fall, is not a necessary condition of free action." Here DeGrazia's assertion is simply off target. Freedom to fall is not the same as "ability to act otherwise". DeGrazia rightly says, "My inability to stab or shoot a loved one or innocent person is due to my stable values and preferences."[8] We are free to fall where we are free to acquire, or decline to acquire, for reasons, "values and preferences" which may become stable by being tested and proving to be effective, among other things, in making the world a better place. Here DeGrazia takes a line similar to that of Tom Douglas.[9] My quarrel is with the process whereby those apparent values and preferences are acquired and become stable, and my purpose is to try to enable those who acquire them to be free to continue to test them by seeing whether holding them does indeed conduce to the good. I say "apparent" values and preferences because pro-social attitudes are attributed "backwards" so to speak by looking at the way people act and inferring their values.[10] The label

---

[8] DeGrazia, "Moral Enhancement, Freedom, and What We (Should) Value in Moral Behaviour", p. 366.

[9] Tom Douglas, "Moral Enhancement via Direct Emotion Modulation: A Reply to John Harris", *Bioethics*, vol. 27, no. 3 (2013): 160–8.

[10] Molly J. Crockett, Luke Clark, Marc D. Hauser, and Trevor W. Robbins, "Serotonin Selectively Influences Moral Judgment and Behavior through Effects on Harm Aversion", *Proceedings of the National Academy of Sciences of the United States of America*, vol. 107, no. 40 (2010): 17433–8; Molly J. Crockett, Luke Clark, Marc D. Hauser, and Trevor W. Robbins, "Reply to Harris and Chan: Moral Judgment is More than Rational Deliberation", *Proceedings of the National Academy of Sciences of the United States of America*, vol. 107, no. 50 (2010): E184.

"pro-social" is then given to the interpretation of behaviour. My problem is that behaviour that may be "pro-social" in the sense that it is expressive of concern for the well-being of those by whom the agent is actually confronted, may actually be anti-social in larger context, when account is taken of the greater good that might have been done by choosing a different strategy which is calculated to do more good to more people; perhaps people who are out of sight and therefore out of mind, except to a reflective moral consciousness.[11]

The issue is whether or not someone who, like Martin Luther, says honestly "here I stand, I can do no other" is able to ask themselves whether this psychological fact (if it is one) is or is not morally regrettable. It is interesting how seductive this sort of pseudo destiny is. Marianne Faithfull recently followed Martin Luther by remarking "I recently looked at my Austrian-Hungarian family tree—my great-great-uncle Leopold von Sacher-Masoch, Venus in Furs and all that. I don't think I had any choice really, but to be very decadent."[12] The freedom of which I (and I believe Milton) speak, the freedom to fall, is the freedom to decide whether or not to fall for reasons which have to do with what is best "all things considered". Anything which by influencing attitudes or emotional responses inhibits that ability significantly, is inimical to freedom. I am not suggesting that BM necessarily always has this effect, only that methods so far advanced by neuroscientists and some philosophers of neuroscience do seem inevitably to have this effect.[13]

My claim is that someone whom MB has made incapable of choosing to "stab or shoot someone who was trying to kill a loved one or an innocent person, if no less violent means of protection were available" has lost the freedom to make moral choices and this is what I fear may be the result of MB that inhibits the ability to do violence where morally

[11] Chan and Harris, "Moral Enhancement and Pro-Social Behaviour"; John Harris and Sarah Chan, "Moral Behavior is Not What It Seems", *Proceedings of the National Academy of Sciences of the United States of America*, vol. 107, no. 50 (2010): E183; Anna Pacholczyk, "Moral Enhancement: What is It and Do We Want It?", *Law, Innovation and Technology*, vol. 3, no. 2 (2011): 251–77.

[12] Dave Simpson, "Marianne Faithfull: 'I don't think I had any choice but to be decadent'", *The Guardian*, 10 January 2013: <http://www.guardian.co.uk/culture/2013/jan/10/marianne-faithfull-decadent-mick-jagger>, accessed 26 January 2015.

[13] Crockett et al., "Serotonin Selectively Influences Moral Judgment and Behavior"; Crockett et al., "Reply to Harris and Chan"; Patricia Churchland, *Braintrust* (Princeton and Oxford: Princeton University Press, 2011).

appropriate. In conceding that he "could probably stab or shoot someone who was trying to kill a loved one" DeGrazia is conceding my point entirely. Of course whether he could or not is an empirical question and we may hope neither he nor I are ever tested. My concern is that there seems to be a real possibility that certain forms of MB will radically reduce that probability with disastrous results. I could of course be wrong, but so could DeGrazia. What I am not wrong about, I believe, is defending a viable and indeed fairly common sense (not that that is much of a recommendation!) view of when it is appropriate to say that freedom has been lost. Not of course totally lost, but lost to an extent that is inimical to liberty understood in the way, for example, that Mill interpreted it.[14]

DeGrazia says "we should not exaggerate the value of freedom". I agree, just as we should not exaggerate anything; exaggeration is, after all, distortion. But in this final flourish DeGrazia fails to distinguish a concept of morality properly so called from a policy of harm reduction by non-moral means, by the administration of a molecule that reduces aggressiveness indiscriminately, but which, as I have argued,[15] because of that may also reduce the sort of aggressiveness that leads people to defend themselves and others.

If, for example, we deploy a policy of the preventive detention of people from socio-economic or ethnic groups which are disproportionately highly represented in criminal convictions, but who have not committed any crime, we may reduce crime and make society safer in a sense. But freedom is thereby radically compromised and few would judge such a course to be a moral enhancement. Although the analogy is not exact (as this exchange between DeGrazia and I demonstrates) it illustrates at least the structure of three important dimensions of my stance on MB. The first is that a decrease in behaviour that causes harm to others may look as though it makes the world a better place but it is unlikely to change people's moral outlook or judgements, although what happens certainly changes what they are able to do, or more modestly, what they are likely to do. Second and more important, the resulting

[14] John Stuart Mill, *On Liberty*. In Mary Warnock (ed.), *Utilitarianism* (London: Collins Fontana, 1962), pp. 126–251.

[15] Harris, "Moral Enhancement and Freedom"; Harris, "Moral Progress and Moral Enhancement"; Harris, "What It's Like to be Good"; Harris, "'Ethics is for Bad Guys!': Putting the 'Moral' into Moral Enhancement"; Chan and Harris, "Moral Enhancement and Pro-Social Behaviour".

diminution in the liberty of those affected has not been factored in to the effects either of a penal policy of preventive detention or of a social policy of biological manipulation. Finally and most important by far, there is reason to believe that increases in pro-sociality may not effect a morally better outcome "all things considered" precisely because they reduce the ability of agents to consider all things.[16]

5.1 The All-Female World

To conclude, I do not think that chemical or molecular moral enhancement is unethical or even wrong-headed per se, nor do I think, for example, that our current average serotonin or oxytocin levels are necessarily optimal. What I have severe reservations about is the use of e.g. Citalopram and other SSRIs to prevent individuals from making less pro-social choices, but possibly more ethical choices.

Rather than tinkering with chemicals or molecules which influence attitudes and emotions I would recommend that the most effective and ethical moral enhancer so far available is learning to subject emotional reactions to the scrutiny of reason. In short I take moral enhancement to involve enhancing our ability to think ethically (cognitive enhancement), not manipulating the probability of some people reacting in ways that *others* deem ethical.

It may be instructive to conclude by reconsidering a scenario I developed thirty years ago[17] as one possibility with a robust evidence base, for effecting moral enhancement by non-invasive methods. This scenario involves taking seriously the ethical advantages of creating an all-female society or even an all-female world and what might constitute reasons for effecting this or its equivalent. Consider, women are widely believed to be less aggressive and, statistics demonstrate, far less likely to be convicted of criminal behaviour or otherwise culpably involved with the criminal justice system than are men.[18] One prospect that might

---

[16] Harris, "What It's Like to be Good".

[17] In this section I deploy again a scenario I first developed in my book *The Value of Life*, pp. 166–74.

[18] *Statistics on Women and the Criminal Justice System 2013*. A Ministry of Justice publication under Section 95 of the Criminal Justice Act 1991. Available at: <https://www.gov.uk/government/uploads/system/uploads/attachment_data/file/380090/women-cjs-2013.pdf>, accessed 27 June 2015. I assume that similar results would hold true for many or most other jurisdictions.

rationally be judged to constitute moral enhancement might be the radical feminization of men; another might be the creation of an all-female society or world.

Suppose, as I wrote in 1985,[19] that it were possible for women to reproduce without men and to produce thereby only females. The development of efficient and safe parthenogenetic reproduction might be one method; another might be by reprogramming human cells, perhaps fibroblasts, to become female totipotent cells; a third might be human cloning.

Suppose, further, that these advances coincided with the resurgence of a particularly vigorous and militant feminism, a feminism which believed that a good measure of the evils of the world had been brought about both by the dominance of men, and by the dominance of certain distinctively (though not exclusively) male characteristics. Suppose they believed that men were on the whole more egocentric, aggressive, competitive, and intolerant than women, and that these features made them in turn more violent, insensitive, and perhaps more callous. It might then seem a rational and progressive step to attempt to create a society from which these disastrous characteristics, and the characters that possessed them, had been eliminated. It would not of course matter that these gender differences could be established beyond doubt, what would matter would be that women on the whole accepted the validity of these differences. What matters for our exemplary purposes is that most women see the circumstances in which they find themselves as making both highly desirable and urgent the establishment of a radically new sort of society, a society in which the human defects that were leading so apparently inexorably to disaster might be eliminated or at least minimized. It might well seem, both to feminists and perhaps to women generally, that it was men and male dominance that had brought these disasters to the world. If so, they might wish to create a society in which men had no part, not because, like women in the past, they would be relegated to the role of second-class citizens, but rather because they would simply not be there.

The rationale of this society might be the simple proposition that reform required not the development, acceptance, and implementation

---

[19] For the remainder of this chapter, as indicated, I borrow liberally from my earlier book.

of a new political and moral theory, but rather required a new type of citizen. And the society which produced such citizens would be founded on, and embody, not a political so much as, say, a eugenic theory. Indeed our hypothetical radicals might as easily have been influenced by the doomsday scenario imagined by Persson and Savulescu and criticized elsewhere in this book.

One of the fears most commonly expressed about attempts to change the human personality, for example by genetic engineering, by moral or indeed by chemical and molecular agents that enhance pro-sociality, what Persson and Savulescu refer to as methods of "moral bioenhancement" is simply, as I also claim in this book, that we cannot predict what other undesirable changes would be consequent on such an attempt.

Now in proposing an all-female society, we would not be faced with quite the same problems. For one thing we know (roughly perhaps in the case of men) what women are like. We would not be contemplating the creation of new or radically altered human beings, merely the eventual elimination of men.

This long (and statistically highly significant) experience in healthy human subjects of what the effects of being a woman are on actual women would give the experiment a sound scientific basis. It would give women a good reason to think that an all-female society would be a change for the better.

Of course such a brave new world would have its drawbacks. We may, however, be inclined to exaggerate these. The first and most obvious disadvantage is that the men wouldn't like it (which invites the obvious, and not entirely frivolous, retort that the men aren't going to get it!). It is whether or not the women would like it that is the question at issue. I would like to think that they would miss us, and find the prospect of a society and a life without men wholly unappealing. But I wouldn't want to bet my life on it. Certainly women would in the future have to face the prospect of adapting their sexuality, and their breeding and child-rearing patterns, to substantially altered circumstances. But they might, and we'll suppose they will, find the prospect of the gains more alluring than the prospect of the losses is depressing, that what they'll lose on the swings is more than compensated for by the gains on the roundabouts.

Part of the viability of the emergence of an all-female society will depend on the way it is to be achieved. It would be hard to claim that the brave new world that would not have such people in it would have a good claim to constitute the moral progress it was designed to achieve if it could only be brought about literally over the dead bodies of men. However, we can imagine one way in which the women in our imagined circumstances might go about planning the creation of their new society. Let's also suppose that they are convinced and agreed that if a morally respectable plan can be worked out they will implement it.

We can suppose that the women in our imagined society are as sensitive, generous, and morally scrupulous as their ideals lead us to expect. They believe that the transition should be gradual, and as painless to men (but not of course to male egos) as it is possible to make it. They resolve that the best way of achieving the new society is simply to let men gradually die out. Until they become extinct through non-replacement, the women will go on treating them exactly (as far as possible) as before. They will continue to associate with men on the same basis, everything will be as it was, except that women will resolutely refuse to allow children to be born other than by methods which exclude the possibility of male offspring. In the transition period men will initially notice little change. The women, being both exceptionally resolute and exceptionally kind-hearted, agree to maintain their existing relationships with men and further agree that men can go on ruling and managing and dominating and so on to their hearts' content. There's no reason why the women should not, if they wish, continue to sleep with men, and being kind-hearted perhaps they will (as a sort of consolation prize awarded to men to help them bear the thought of their final redundancy?).

Men can do everything they used to do except father children. And of course they never had a moral nor yet even a legal right to do this against the wishes of women. In this respect also things will be as they always were.

Of course the people born into the new society will not be the same ones that would have been born had the idea never been floated, but this will be true of any society in which people vary their breeding habits from generation to generation. If, for example, people begin to breed later rather than sooner, then the children born will not be those who would have been born had this change not taken place. And of course choices of partner and of month of conception also create different people than those who would have been born had these factors been different.

As men die out and the feminist millennium approaches, women will gradually take over all positions previously occupied by men. Traditional family life will change. It may cease altogether and be replaced by collective child-rearing and extended families. Some women will certainly set up sexual partnerships, and rear children in the traditional two-'parent' unit. Some others will find the possibility of having children without sexual relationships a distinct plus. Others presumably will find the loss of heterosexual relationships a severe source of unhappiness. However, all agree that this prospect, however bleak (or cheerful), is distinctly preferable to the alternative, the old male-dominated and disaster-prone society, and agree that the prospective gains are well worth the foreseen losses.

Suppose that interplanetary travel eventually revealed to us a world very much like our own, inhabited by beings of one gender who reproduced parthenogenetically. Suppose further that they were very like female human beings. If their world proved to be one in which wars and violence were unknown or rare, in which the people coexisted without the need for competition and aggression and were reasonably happy and contented into the bargain, it is not obvious that we would find their world wholly deplorable nor manifestly inferior to our own. If on further inquiry we found that they did have pleasurable physical, as well as emotional, relationships with one another, we might well even come to admire their world and wish, wistfully, that we were able to emulate it. It might well be not unreasonable or fanciful to conclude that the gains might well be worth the losses, if only we could repeat the experiment here.

Finally and crucially, we have no reason to think that human women are less free than their male counterparts, except of course where male domination has brought this about. We therefore have reasons to be complacent that such a scenario as the feminization of men or the creation of an all-female world would, at least from the perspective of its effects on liberty, be relatively unproblematic. What other reasons there might be to object to such an experiment I leave for readers to consider.

If for example Persson and Savulescu are right when they claim: "in order for the majority of citizens of liberal democracies to be willing to go along with the constraints on their extravagant consumption, their moral motivation will have to be enhanced"[20] and if the feminization of men or

---

[20] Ingmar Persson and Julian Savulescu, *Unfit for the Future* (Oxford: Oxford University Press, 2012), p. 2.

the creation of an all-female world offers just such a prospect, I assume that they, at least, will be receptive to the moral possibilities of the scenario just reconsidered, particularly when they consider that the research evidence in its favour is considerably more robust than that available for what they call moral bioenhancement.[21]

[21] I wish to thank Anna Pacholczyk and Sadie Regmi for very useful and detailed comments on this chapter.

6

The God Machine, the God Delusion, and the Death of Liberty

From "The Unknown Citizen"— W. H. Auden
(To JS/07 M 378 This Marble Monument Is Erected by the State)
...Our researchers into Public Opinion are content
That he held the proper opinions for the time of year;
When there was peace, he was for peace: when there was war,
he went.
He was married and added five children to the population,
Which our Eugenist says was the right number for a parent of his
generation.
And our teachers report that he never interfered with their
education.
Was he free? Was he happy? The question is absurd:
Had anything been wrong, we should certainly have heard.[1]

It is not one man nor a million, but the *spirit* of liberty that must be preserved. The waves which dash upon the shore are, one by one, broken, but the *ocean* conquers nevertheless. It overwhelms the Armada, it wears the rock. In like manner, whatever the struggle of individuals, the great cause will gather strength.[2]

Lord Byron, Ravenna Journal, 11 January 1821, pp. 163–4

Verres deliberately chose a spot within sight if Italy (for the execution of Gavius) so that Gavius, while dying in dreadful agony, might appreciate how narrow the strait was that separated freedom from slavery, and that Italy might see her own son nailed to a cross, and

---

[1] <http://www.poets.org/viewmedia.php/prmMID/15549#sthash.kWhaw9GK.dpuf>.
[2] Quoted by Iris Origo, *The Last Attachment: The Story of Byron and Teresa Guiccioli* (New York: Books and Co/Helen Marx Books, 2000), p. xxvi.

paying the most terrible and extreme punishment that can be inflicted on slaves.

Cicero, *In Verrem* II.5[3]

W. H. Auden's "unknown citizen" is the perfect model for the citizens of a molecularly morally enhanced society in that he cannot even think of acting independently—for the unknown citizen the idea of independent thought is literally unthinkable. Auden's critique is implicit in the description he gives, just as the habit of conformity is intrinsic to the unknown citizen's of Auden's imagined state. For Auden the citizen of which he speaks and whose life he ironically memorializes, could never imagine the need to defend liberty because he has been rendered incapable of understanding in what it might consist. Byron disembodies liberty, identifying it as a spirit, an idea, which humans understand and can exemplify even when their individual struggle for freedom founders. Cicero's admiration for Gavius stems from his passionate republicanism. The spirit of his prosecution of Verres, the tyrant of Sicily, and its appeal to the laws of the republic he loved, eventually foundered in truly Byronic style on the rocks of another vicious tyrant, Mark Antony. But more than Antony or Brutus, it is Cicero's courage in defence of liberty that makes him, if not "the noblest Roman of them all"[4] as Shakespeare's Mark Antony said of Brutus, at least the one most worthy of emulation.

A crucial issue both in the understanding of the nature of morality and for that reason also in the analysis of what might count as moral enhancement is the role of, indeed the nature of, moral decision-making. Various devices have been from time to time deployed to break the link between thought and action, to show that decisions are not an essential part of the way in which humans connect with the world and hence that responsibility attaches to choices rather than to actions. In this chapter we examine further one such attempt and note that while thought and

---

[3] The strait referred to is the Strait of Messina which separates Sicily and Italy where Gavius of Consa, a Roman citizen, had invoked protection of the law by repeatedly saying, as he was being tortured and executed, "I am a Roman Citizen". This incantation by law and tradition protected Roman citizens throughout the Empire from ill usage. Cicero, *Political Speeches*, trans. H. D. Berry (Oxford: Oxford University Press, 2006), p. 94.

[4] William Shakespeare, *Julius Caesar*, Act 5, Scene 5. Brutus is addressing Cassius. The Arden Shakespeare, *Complete Works*, ed. Richard Proudfoot, Ann Thomson, and David Scott Kastan (Walton-on-Thames: Thomas Nelson and Sons, 1998).

action can be sundered they remain, paradoxically perhaps, inextricably linked in ways that inform our understanding of freedom.

In Chapter 4, I took as one point of departure Ingmar Persson and Julian Savulescu's paper on a related theme.[5] In that paper they summarize part of their argument as follows:

With the progress of science, which would be speeded up by cognitive enhancement it becomes increasingly possible for small groups of people, or even single individuals, to cause great harms to millions of people.

. . . it is enough if very few of us are malevolent or vicious enough to use this power for all of us to run an unacceptable increase of the risk of death and disaster. To eliminate this risk, cognitive enhancement would have to be accompanied by a *moral* enhancement which extends to *all* of us, since such moral enhancement could reduce malevolence. . . . That is, safe, effective moral enhancement would be compulsory.[6]

If Julian and Ingmar really wish to leave space for freedom then we agree, but I don't believe it for a moment, for reasons we are about to consider.

Some of the mischief is in the meaning . . . in this case of the words "safe and effective" moral enhancement. I have never been opposed to moral enhancement per se. Despite persistent suggestions from Ingmar and Julian to the contrary my entire effort has been directed to the meaning of moral enhancement and to the issues of safety (including moral; and political safety—more of which anon) and efficacy.

Let us now come up to date. Ingmar and Julian have made two recent further clarifications of their position and they reject my concerns about it. First in their recent book *Unfit for the Future*[7] and subsequently in their "Moral Enhancement, Freedom and the God Machine".[8]

Before turning to the horrific God Machine, let's start with their more modest claims in *Unfit for the Future*.

---

[5] Ingmar Persson and Julian Savulescu, "The Perils of Cognitive Enhancement and the Urgent Imperative to Enhance the Moral Character of Humanity", *Journal of Applied Philosophy*, vol. 25, no. 3 (2008): 162–77.

[6] Persson and Savulescu, "The Perils of Cognitive Enhancement", p. 166.

[7] Ingmar Persson and Julian Savulescu, *Unfit for the Future: The Need for Moral Enhancement* (Oxford: Oxford University Press, 2012).

[8] Julian Savulescu and Ingmar Persson, "Moral Enhancement, Freedom and the God Machine", *The Monist*, vol. 95, no. 3 (2012): 399–421. Available at: <http://www.ncbi.nlm.nih.gov/pmc/articles/PMC3431130/pdf/ukmss-49380.pdf>, accessed 11 June 2015.

Harris's core claim about freedom, expressed in the idiom of Milton's *Paradise Lost*, seems to be that 'sufficiency to stand is worthless, literally morally bankrupt, without freedom to fall'. In other words, a decision to act in a way that is morally right is morally worthless—meaning presumably that you are not morally praiseworthy for it—if you are not free not to make the decision.[9]

Julian and Ingmar's presumptions here are, well . . . presumptuous. I am talking about freedom, not about the state of the soul of the agent. What is morally important here is to be actually free, what is morally bankrupt is the illusion of freedom.

Julian and Ingmar then produce an example of Harry Frankfurt. Here it is:

Imagine that you decide to do the morally right thing on the basis of considering reasons for and against, as somebody who is morally responsible is supposed to do. Imagine, however, that there is a freaky mechanism in your brain which would have kicked in if you had been in the process of making not this decision, but a decision to do something which is morally wrong . . . Hence you are not free to fall . . . Would the presence of this freaky mechanism mean that you are not praiseworthy for making the right decision? It is hard to see why it would: after all the mechanism was never called into operation; it remained idle. In fact you decided to do the morally right thing for precisely the same reasons as someone whose brain does not feature the freaky mechanism could [sic] do, and whose praiseworthiness is therefore not in doubt.[10]

This is the famous "locked house". If you were shut into a locked house which you could never leave, but did not know that all the doors and windows were impassable and as a matter of fact never formed the desire even to think of leaving, or to try to leave, would you be free? Well you certainly would not be free to leave, and prison is normally considered the antithesis of freedom. Frankfurt possibly, and Julian and Ingmar certainly, are ignoring the distinction between being capable and not being thwarted or frustrated. The person with the freaky mechanism is not thwarted or frustrated if they never make the decision which will be blocked but they do not have either freedom of decision-making, or of action. There is an analogy here with disability. The person born blind will never attempt to look at pictures or TV, certain courses of action are futile, they likewise do not have freedom of choice or action with respect

---

[9] Persson and Savulescu, *Unfit for the Future*, p. 114.
[10] Persson and Savulescu, *Unfit for the Future*, p. 114.

to accessing visual experiences. If the blinding was deliberate we would judge them to have been rendered less free than they might have been if sighted but because they do not know what it's like to see things they will (possibly) not feel thwarted by their inability.

The issue is not praiseworthiness, it is liberty. Julian and Ingmar conclude: "freedom of will or action is not indispensable for moral responsibility. So Harris's 'freedom to fall' is not essential for moral choice and action."[11] But I am talking precisely about moral responsibility, that is responsibility for the actions, the doings, the effects that are part of our moral decision-making. If the decision-making part of the process is separable from the actions upon which we decide, then what is the agent responsible for? Agents are quintessentially actors; to be an agent is to be capable of action. Without agency in this sense, decision-making is, as I claimed and continue to claim, morally and indeed practically barren—literally without issue!

Decisions to no effect are pointless from the moral perspective; for what is a good state of mind worth, if it makes no difference to the world. At best Julian and Ingmar can say "Harris's 'freedom to fall' is not essential for moral choice". They cannot say as they do that "Harris's 'freedom to fall' is not essential for moral choice *and action*".

Frankfurt's freaky mechanism would soon impact on the freedom and hence the moral responsibility of agents. Whole classes of choices would never be made and as a result the individual would be a different sort of being, constituted by the choices they habitually made. It is not credible that a person in a locked house would never try the doors and windows nor that a normal human being would never in the course of their lives make choices that the freaky mechanism would block. Thank God Adam listened to his wife and she to the serpent or the world would be as morally bankrupt as heaven.

This interestingly would, if Julian and Ingmar or indeed Frankfurt are right, constitute the definitive refutation of the idea that "ought implies can". We need to remember that conclusions about what ought to be done can be said to ourselves as well as to others, but if we cannot follow our own imperatives then our imperatives are, as I have said, pointless.

---

[11]   Persson and Savulescu, *Unfit for the Future*, p. 115.

Consider, there are two principles in play here: PAP (the principle of alternative possibilities) and OiC (Ought implies Can). Then

1. OiC is incompatible with determinism (of whatever kind) and
2. Indeterminism implies PAP (that one can do other than what has been determined by the freaky mechanism or, as we will see later, by the God Machine).
   Then
3. Denying PAP also involves denying OiC.

Frankfurt's freaky mechanism shows that for those cursed with the mechanism there are not alternative possibilities even though they believe there are.[12]

6.1 Responsibility, Autonomy, and Moral Decision-Making—A Pertinent Digression

Decisions are decisive, that's why we make them! It is also why we are responsible for them and for their consequences; our responsibility stems from our will, from the fact that we did these things on purpose. Some believe, however, that either the discoveries of neuroscience or the innovation, and the products to which innovation leads, are undermining both our responsibility and our autonomy and demonstrating that freedom to choose or free will is an illusion. It is important to know whether this is so and if it is, the extent to which our autonomy and its consequent responsibility are threatened, and whether ultimately such threats, if they exist, are to be feared or welcomed. This is partly the subject of this chapter.

To understand this better we need to start further back and consider some fundamental concepts which inform this debate.

---

[12] I am grateful to Michael Quante for helping me to be clear about what is at stake here. This is of course question-begging concerning the compatibilism–incompatibilism debate. Those who want to avoid this and leave open the possibility that a compatibilist reading of OiC is possible, cannot say that denying PAP logically entails denying OiC. See also Michael Quante, "Autonomy for Real People", in Christopher Lumer and Sando Nannini (eds.), *Intentionality, Deliberation and Autonomy* (Aldershot: Ashgate, 2007), pp. 209–26.

Autonomy, the ability to choose freely and the *responsibility*, or the consequences of choice, which it entails are two key concepts. Autonomy is literally "self-government" and it is a commonplace that government, including self-government, the exercise of power and responsibility in the interests of the individual or the state, can teach us much about our place in and our effect on the world.

Democracies, for example, exercise the power of the people on their behalf, in their interests and for their protection. To do this a government makes decisions, to intervene or not to intervene, to put in protections against disaster or not to do so and each decision, to act or to refrain, makes a difference. If it doesn't there would be no point in making it. All this is impossible without genuine choice.

Such decisions include mechanisms to prevent, mitigate, or respond to the effects of fire, famine, flood, disease or injury, crime, foreign invasion or internal terror. We can all see why such decisions are necessary and what turns on making the right choice. Governments are responsible then in two senses. They are vested with the responsibility to act on our behalf and they are responsible, that is accountable, for the ways in which these decisions are made and for their effects.

It is the same with individuals: we have responsibility for ourselves and our decisions, our deliberate actions or refrainings, and we are responsible in the second sense identified here, that is we are accountable for our decisions and their effects, accountable in short for the way we govern ourselves and for the effects of so doing.

But this second sense of responsibility, namely accountability, is predicated on the idea that our decisions are our own, are expressions of our will, and not merely the products of brute forces, whether natural, social, or divine. In short, it assumes that there is genuine power to choose behind both governance and self-governance.

On this view each decision is world changing and world creating. The world will be a different place to the extent that something is decided and to the extent to which that decision makes a difference. That is why decision-making matters; each decision is, in effect, a choice between possible worlds made actual by that decision. And of course while every event is also world changing, decisions are special because the decision, the choice by a consciousness, is what makes the difference.

Decisions then are not only world creating, they are self-defining. We are the product of our past decisions; they are in large part responsible for making us what we are: our history and our future is defined by them. We are the persons we make of ourselves.[13]

Of course our decisions have antecedents which exercise causal effects; they are part of the complex causal chain which precedes every event. Some of these antecedents are chemical, neurological, or biological, others are social: peer example and pressure, education, knowledge, including knowledge of cause and effect. Still other influences include previous acts of the will, previous decisions which have made us the individuals that we are.

At the Diet of Worms on 18 April 1521, Martin Luther famously defended his principles thus:

> Unless I am convinced by proofs from Scriptures or by plain and clear reasons and arguments, I can and will not retract, for it is neither safe nor wise to do anything against conscience. Here I stand. I can do no other. God help me. Amen.[14]

He was not, as is sometimes said, acting involuntarily, not literally able to "do no other". As he himself says, he was acting for what he perceived to be "clear reasons and arguments", exercising his will in the light of these and like any rational creature "compelled" by reason and force of argument along with all the other antecedent causes but not excluded

---

[13] For more on autonomy and responsibility see H. L. A. Hart, *Punishment and Responsibility* (Oxford: Clarendon Press, 1968), Chapter IX, Postscript; Jonathan Glover, *Responsibility* (London: Routledge & Kegan Paul, 1970); D. F. Pears (ed.), *Freedom and the Will* (London: Macmillan, 1969); Gerald Dworkin, *The Theory and Practice of Autonomy* (Cambridge: Cambridge University Press, 1988); Onora O'Neill, *Autonomy and Trust in Bioethics* (Cambridge: Cambridge University Press, 2002); Joseph Raz, *The Morality of Freedom* (Oxford: Clarendon Press, 1986); Jeremy Waldron, "Moral Autonomy and Personal Autonomy", in John Christman and Joel Anderson (eds.), *Autonomy and the Challenges to Liberalism* (Cambridge: Cambridge University Press, 2005), pp. 307–29; John Harris, *The Value of Life* (London: Routledge, 1985), Chapters 10 and 11; and John Harris, *Violence and Responsibility* (London: Routledge & Kegan Paul, 1980).

[14] I cannot remember where I found the lines quoted in the text; there are many extant versions but I prefer them to one of the many alternative formulations, namely: "Luther then replied: Your Imperial Majesty and Your Lordships demand a simple answer. Here it is, plain and unvarnished. Unless I am convicted [convinced] of error by the testimony of Scripture or (since I put no trust in the unsupported authority of Pope or councils, since it is plain that they have often erred and often contradicted themselves) by manifest reasoning, I stand convicted [convinced] by the Scriptures to which I have appealed, and my conscience is taken captive by God's word, I cannot and will not recant anything, for to act against our conscience is neither safe for us, nor open to us. On this I take my stand. I can do no other. God help me." <http://www-personal.ksu.edu/~lyman/english233/Luther-Diet_of_Worms.htm>.

by those causes. But this sort of compulsion is at the heart of autonomy; self-government is pointless (as well as non-existent) if not exercisable.

Of course reasons and arguments are powerful causes of decisions and of actions; they are also often satisfying explanations of what we say and do; if they were not, we would not seek for them and deploy them in explanation and defence of our decisions. Such things have a crucial role in the chain of causation, or in the explanation, of action.

The issue of course is whether or not they leave room for an exercise of will, and if they do, whether something else has a determining effect on our decisions such that, while feeling free and authentic in the exercise of our decision-making, such a feeling must be considered, in fact, an illusion.

If it is an illusion it is one that has immense social and psychological power and one also that has crucial legal and administrative convenience. We will clearly be reluctant to abandon all of these things. The question for neuroscience is as to whether there is any compelling reason or set of arguments to lead us to suppose that we might have to abandon what so many feel to be their precious and vital freedom. And if there is, neuroscience will also have to explain why it is not the reasons or the arguments that are operative but something else, something perhaps rather more physical or chemical. These reasons are what the God Machine is designed to provide, but they are illusory.

As I have noted earlier in this book, in Book III of *Paradise Lost*[15] John Milton reports God as saying to his "Only begotten Son" that if man is perverted by the "false guile" of Satan he has only himself to blame:

> whose fault?
> Whose but his own? Ingrate, he had of me
> All he could have; I made him just and right,
> Sufficient to have stood, though free to fall.[16]

Here Milton is expressing a thought similar to that of Luther. The sufficiency to have stood is man's ability to explain and justify his choices in terms which fully account for and explain his actions. Milton has God choosing under the constraint of logic, just as did Luther, for without

---

[15] John Milton, *Paradise Lost*, ed. John Leonard (London: Penguin Books, 2000). Milton first published *Paradise Lost* in 1667.

[16] Milton, *Paradise Lost*, lines 96ff.

that freedom there is no virtue in right action and no evil in wrongdoing. Milton saw that God was bound by things outside his or her will but present to his or her reason: "he had of me all he could have".

Once choice is divorced from action it is morally bankrupt and indeed I don't think it coherent to speak of choice in this way for any practical purpose. Once thought and action are divorced in this way it is difficult to keep a grip on reality.

Frankfurt's freaky mechanism is a form of "behaviour control". It would, if it actually existed, have prevented any one who possessed it from learning from moral mistakes and so would have caused them to lose, and hence never learn from, the role our choices play for all of us in creating our own characteristics. If we didn't see the consequences of bad decisions how would we learn from them? The freaky mechanism would attack agency itself not just prevent bad decisions. Neither Frankfurt nor Persson and Savulescu have really thought this example through.

It is, I am afraid, one of those absurd philosophers' examples which, in Wittgenstein's words, are of no effect; "a wheel that can be turned though nothing else moves with it, is not part of the mechanism".[17] Frankfurt's freaky mechanism disconnects thought from action and so changes the very nature of both and hence the nature of what it means to have thoughts like that and the meaning of doing things like that. It is this divorce of thought and action and indeed thought and reality that gets philosophy a bad name.

Which pertinent digression brings us to Experience Machines.

6.1.1 Experience machines

There is an analogy here between Frankfurt's example and the God Machine to which we will turn in a moment on the one hand and Robert Nozick[18] and Jonathan Glover's[19] discussion of Experience Machines and Dreamworlds on the other.

In Nozick's Experience Machine people feel as if things are actually happening to them but the reality is that they only have the experience of

[17] Ludwig Wittgenstein, *Philosophical Investigations*, trans G. E. M. Anscombe (Oxford: Basil Blackwell, 1968), para. 271.

[18] Robert Nozick, *Anarchy, State and Utopia* (Oxford: Basil Blackwell, 1974), pp. 42ff.

[19] Jonathan Glover, *What Sort of People Should There Be?* (Harmondsworth: Penguin Books, 1984), Chapters 5, 6, and 7.

it happening created by brain stimulation. Nozick asks "What does matter to us in addition to our experiences?" and he answers that "we want to *be* a certain way, to be a certain sort of person".[20] The clear suggestion is that what seems is not enough. Hamlet himself, in his famous riposte to his mother makes a similar point about the significance of the difference between appearance and reality: "Seems, madam? Nay it is. I know not 'seems'."[21]

Glover imagines a "dreamworld" in which we can choose to experience (though not to live) a range of possible lives. In a wide-ranging discussion which is highly relevant to freedom and to authenticity he concludes *inter alia* that consideration of:

[T]he dreamworld sets limits to the kinds of possible improvements over our ordinary world. This can be seen by asking the question whether people in the dreamworld would be able to act in ways that harm each other. If the answer is 'no', we are back with the drawbacks of behaviour control. We have lost a large range of possible choices, and have correspondingly lost some of the role our choices play in creating our own characteristics. (Being considerate, for instance, would no longer be a characteristic we could freely choose from among other possibilities.)[22]

Dreamworlds are, like Frankfurt's freaky mechanism, a form of behaviour control that purports to disconnect thought from action. This disconnect is very important and we will return to it as we consider now another loose cog in a very shaky machine—the God Machine.

6.1.2 Obliterating immoral behaviour: the God Machine

This is how Julian and Ingmar[23] set out their great thought experiment and it is ingenious and deserves our full attention:

The Great Moral Project was completed in 2045. This involved construction of the most powerful, self-learning, self-developing bioquantum computer ever constructed called the God Machine. The God Machine would monitor the thoughts, beliefs, desires and intentions of every human being. It was capable of modifying these within nanoseconds, without the conscious recognition by any human subjects.

---

[20] Nozick, *Anarchy, State and Utopia*, p. 43.

[21] William Shakespeare, *Hamlet*, Act 1, Scene 2. The Arden Shakespeare.

[22] Glover, *What Sort of People Should There Be?*, p. 103.

[23] Savulescu and Persson, "Moral Enhancement, Freedom and the God Machine", <http://www.ncbi.nlm.nih.gov/pmc/articles/PMC3431130/pdf/ukmss-49380.pdf>, p. 10.

The God Machine was designed to give human beings near complete freedom. It only ever intervened in human action to prevent great harm, injustice or other deeply immoral behaviour from occurring. For example, murder of innocent people no longer occurred. As soon as a person formed the intention to murder, and it became inevitable that this person would act to kill, the God Machine would intervene. The would-be murderer would 'change his mind.' The God Machine would not intervene in trivial immoral acts, like minor instances of lying or cheating. It was only when a threshold insult to some sentient being's interests was crossed would the God Machine exercise its almighty power.

It is important to be clear that the "God Machine" is not a thought experiment or rather not simply a thought experiment. It is a metaphor, an analogy, a rhetorical device which seeks to persuade us that seen in this light things are not so bad. But they are!

Julian and Ingmar insist that *Human beings can still autonomously choose to be moral, since if they choose the moral action, the God Machine will not intervene. Indeed, they are free to be moral. They are only unfree to do grossly immoral acts, like killing or raping.* This is Henry Ford's famous freedom to choose the colour of a model "T": "You can have any colour you like so long as it's black!" Even those who want a black car have no choice, although they get what they want they had no choice. But it is also problematic in another way.

6.1.3 Context is (almost) all

What makes killing immoral, what makes sexual intercourse rape? These are complex philosophical, ethical, legal, and social questions; they are not scientific questions, at least of the sort to which knowledge of brain states could conceivably reveal answers. The answers, whatever they are, are not to be found in states of the brain, nor even the intentions or motives of the agent, although these are not totally irrelevant. This is why I have consistently opposed the rather silly claims of some neuropsychologists that so-called pro-social attitudes are the stuff of which moral judgements are made.[24]

Wittgenstein famously remarked: "If God had looked into our minds he would not have been able to see there of whom we were speaking."[25]

---

[24] Sarah Chan and John Harris, "Moral Enhancement and Prosocial Behaviour", *Journal of Medical Ethics*, vol. 37, no. 3 (2011): 130–1.

[25] Wittgenstein, *Philosophical Investigations*, Part IIxi at p. 217. Since this is a translation I have taken the liberty of improving upon Elizabeth Anscombe's prose.

Why would he not? Why could he not? The answer is that the ethics of conduct, the answer to questions like: is this murder? or is this rape? are not there to be found.

Think of the concept of grief. Imagine your friend rings at your door, you welcome her in, but she is obviously greatly distressed, ashen faced, trembling and in tears. You ask what the matter is and she tells you that she is suffering the most inconsolable grief. You ask what has happened, what loss has she suffered, who close to her has died and she replies "Oh, no one has died, I have suffered no loss, I am just subject to attacks of grief, a bit like migraine, and I am having a particularly bad attack today."

Why is this incoherent? Obviously because whatever she is experiencing it cannot be grief because the concept of grief involves feelings for and about something independent of her brain, someone who has died. Grief is not the name of a bodily sensation or of the firing of certain neurones, it is not about events in the brain, it is inexorably tied to the events in the world. This is what limits even God's powers of insight in Wittgenstein's remark.

The God Machine might also be programmed or take upon itself the task of regulating self-harm. But consider a recent case, that of a Mexican woman who with a kitchen knife performed a Caesarean section on herself.[26] Or consider an amateur performing emergency surgery at the roadside to try to save a life, a tracheotomy for example? Or the man who attacks someone whom he believes to be a rapist, *in flagrante delicto*, attacking his daughter. Might this father's intentions seem "murderous" to a God Machine? What would his "intentions" look like on the inside seen from the outside? Is this even a sensible question? I myself doubt it, hence my scepticism about much of the so-called work on pro-social or anti-social attitudes and its significance for moral judgements and moral enhancement properly so-called, also my scepticism about the information to be gleaned from considering God Machines.

I could of course be wrong about all this, but I am sceptical about the claims made for moral enhancement and the picture of mind upon which they depend.

---

[26] <http://news.bbc.co.uk/1/hi/health/3606845.stm>, accessed 12 May 2013.

In ethics and law, as well as in biology and neurology, context is hugely important and context is not accessible to the God Machine or even (often) to God herself.

Giuseppe Testa and I wrote, in another context, of a very different example of the importance of context.

In the 90s, scientists defined the genetic hierarchy underlying the development of the eye. The experiment was spectacular, and the very wording in which we still describe its outcome (genetic hierarchy) is a legacy of its seminal character. A single gene, transplanted in tissues of the fly embryo such as the wings and the legs, was able to direct the formation of a whole eye, an ectopic eye. And yet, when the same fly gene was transferred into a mouse to check for its ability to rescue the eyeless mutation that resulted in eye absence, the result remained compelling: again, an eye was formed testifying to the remarkable evolutionary conservation of genes and developmental pathways. But this technological re-enactment of Monod's aphorism 'what is true for E.coli is true for the elephant' also showed that, as expected, a fly gene in the mouse 'forms' a mouse eye. Context, in other words, is just as essential as genes.[27]

This example shows that context is important in biology and may be important in neurology also and that context is not simply bodily or brain context. It may be rash to assume that the God Machine would be capable of understanding the read-out from the brains of her subjects. Just as the sort of eye produced is not only in the gene so the sort of action produced is possibly not only in the neurone.

6.1.4 The good old days

Julian and Ingmar say: *While people weren't free to act immorally in the 'old days' since the law prohibited it on pain of punishment, the install-ment of the God Machine means that it has become literally impossible to do these things.*[28] They imply this is a minor inconvenience at worst. But this is a different level of un-freedom. As with all actions, when we are free, we are only free to do as we like and take the consequences. In the world of the God Machine even this is denied to us; such freedom is "literally impossible".

[27] Giuseppe Testa and John Harris, "Ethics and Synthetic Gametes", *Bioethics*, vol. 19, no. 2 (2005): 146–67.

[28] Savulescu and Persson, "Moral Enhancement, Freedom and the God Machine", <http://www.ncbi.nlm.nih.gov/pmc/articles/PMC3431130/pdf/ukmss-49380.pdf>, p. 11.

In the "old days", *contra* Julian and Ingmar, things were entirely different. Let's just remind ourselves what good old freedom under the law is actually like, the sort of freedom most of us still now enjoy.

In a democratic state under the rule of law there is genuine non-trivial freedom. The government can be (and is) changed at regular, and recently in the UK set, intervals; democratic representatives are account-able to the law and to the people. The operation of the mechanisms of government and the law function in accordance with the constitutionally established and protected consent of the governed; the police and courts can exercise discretion, mitigating circumstances can be considered by the courts, juries can acquit even those who are clearly "guilty" according to the letter of the law (as in many so-called "mercy killing" cases in the UK); civil disobedience can be practised; the state of the law can be, and is, constantly debated and challenged in myriad ways. Most importantly governments can even be changed between elections; leaders can be ousted or, as in the UK lose votes of confidence and have to resign. If Julian and Ingmar cannot see the difference, I literally despair. When they say the "God Machine means that it has become literally impossible to do these things" and imply this is a minor change from the 'old days' when the law prohibited things "on pain of punishment" this seems to me to be some way from reality.

And it gets worse. Talking of the human agent under the operation of the God Machine they say: "It seems to her that she has 'changed her mind' spontaneously – she experiences a life of complete freedom, though she is not free." Denied even the ability to know when our freedom is being curtailed we would lack the motive to rebel and lacking a constitutional and democratic framework for control of the God Machine we would have no recourse whatsoever.

6.2 Censorship

The problem with permitting press and media censorship in any society has always been that once censorship exists citizens have no knowledge of what precisely has been censored and why. They don't know what they don't know. The citizens have no way, even if they approve in principle of certain forms of censorship, of knowing whether or not just the things they would wish to have been prohibited to see or hear or read are the ones that have in fact been banned. That is why liberal democracies view censorship with great suspicion and are vigilant to oppose the handing of such powers to officials, who are naturally inclined to be ... officious. The same goes in spades for the God Machine; once plugged in, the agent only seems to be an agent and will never become aware of the number of times or of the sorts of occasions on which her mind had been changed and so will have no "motive" to withdraw from the machine even if the machine would let them; they also have no way of knowing if the machine has broken down.

And it gets worse even than that:

It is, perhaps, this kind of world which objectors to moral enhancement like Harris fear. Human beings are no longer 'free to fall' or at least not free to fall big time. But it might be wondered what is so bad with such a world after all? Those who value and want to be free can be free, or at least as free as humans can ever be. And everyone is much better off for the absence of evil. There is no physical incarceration or great harm wrought by one human being on another. Why not create the God Machine, as a fail-safe device which kicks in when moral enhancement has not been effective enough?[29]

Do I ask myself "Why not create a God Machine?" You betcha I do! And I answer in the negative. And I do not for a moment think "everyone is much better off for the absence of evil". Or ask myself: "Why not create the God Machine, as a fail-safe device ...?"

The evil would *be* the God Machine itself, a million times worse than Milton's God and how would it be "fail safe"? *Sed quis custodiet ipsos custodes?*—But who guards the guardians? How would the operations of this new megalomaniac be regulated, challenged, or even reviewed?

Julian and Ingmar believe there is "one way in which the God Machine would not compromise autonomy":

Autonomy is the power to make well-grounded, rational decisions and to act in accordance with them. There is one way in which the God Machine would not compromise autonomy, that is, even if it did prevent people from acting immorally. This would be the case if people voluntarily chose to be connected. Voluntarily connecting to the God Machine would then be an example of a precommitment contract, the paradigm example of which is Ulysses and the Sirens.[30]

---

[29] Savulescu and Persson, "Moral Enhancement, Freedom and the God Machine", <http://www.ncbi.nlm.nih.gov/pmc/articles/PMC3431130/pdf/ukmss-49380.pdf>, p. 11.
[30] Savulescu and Persson, "Moral Enhancement, Freedom and the God Machine", <http://www.ncbi.nlm.nih.gov/pmc/articles/PMC3431130/pdf/ukmss-49380.pdf>, p. 11.

This is a poor example and no analogy for the God Machine. Ulysses orders his men to bind him to the mast temporarily and for a particular purpose; his imprisonment has a brief and finite duration and is fully voluntary. It is like agreeing to be sedated for a surgical operation during which one loses the power to say "stop cutting". The proper analogy with the God Machine is selling or giving yourself into slavery, a condition which is open-ended and potentially endless. The rule of the God Machine is literally the rule of a slave-owning tyrant, which, as Julian and Ingmar admit, with magisterial understatement, does "compromise autonomy". The freedom to sell yourself into slavery is, with few exceptions, admitted to be the one exercise of liberty incompatible with the very liberty of which it is claimed to be an instance. Julian and Ingmar have found another. They say: "If there is anything wrong with the God Machine, it seems that at most it is wrong to connect competent adults against their will."[31] But they go on to deny that even this is problematic. "Freedom" they say "is only one value"... "the value of human well-being and respect for the most basic rights outweighs the value of autonomy".[32]

Well this is a point of view... albeit not mine. It may well in the end come down to a clash of values.

But I think what is now clear is that Persson and Savulescu's repeated claims in so many places since I wrote the paper "Moral Enhancement and Freedom" (Chapter 4 of this book) that moral enhancement, as they see it, is not inimical to freedom, are hollow. Moreover my arguments to the effect that both the ways in which moral enhancement is most likely, for the foreseeable future, to function are inimical to freedom and my claims that at least some of their advocates, like Julian and Ingmar, are indeed also inimical to freedom have been shown to be well founded. Some version of the God Machine is, as Persson and Savulescu now admit, what they hope moral enhancement will prove to be. Tragically they think:

Even in those cases in which the God Machine does undermine autonomy, the value of human well being and respect for the most basic rights outweighs the value of Autonomy. This is not controversial. As Mill wrote,

[31] Savulescu and Persson, "Moral Enhancement, Freedom and the God Machine", p. 415.
[32] Savulescu and Persson, "Moral Enhancement, Freedom and the God Machine", p. 416.

"That the only purpose for which power can be rightfully exercised over any member of a civilized community, against his will, is to prevent harm to others. His own good, either physical or moral is not sufficient warrant."

What more moral way to prevent harm to others is there than to cause a person to change his mind?[33]

6.2.1 Libertarians and libertines

This rebuke by Julian and Ingmar to the effect that John Stuart Mill would have approved of the paternalism of the God Machine is not well taken. First autonomy is a basic right quite as much as is freedom from violence or certain levels of well-being. Indeed autonomy (not just the illusion of autonomy) is part of well-being.

We noted earlier them saying: "while people weren't free to act immorally in the 'old days,' since the law prohibited it on pain of punishment, the instalment of the God Machine means that it has become literally impossible to do these things." They imply that the mechanisms of the God Machine are just like, or enough like, the regulation of behaviour effected by laws and regulations that we should accept them as readily or more readily because they are more effective.

Here they fail to recognize a distinction that Mill well understood: that between liberty and licence. Liberty as understood by Mill and indeed as is familiar since Plato, is a moral and political concept, it is an idea, an ideal, and a value. A basic right if ever there was one. Liberty is required for autonomy, literally "self-rule" which is not the same as misrule. Indeed the idea of a "Lord of Misrule" derives from the ancient world and was institutionalized in medieval times.[34] Self-rule, and the liberty it presupposes is as different from licence and the misrule it implies as it is possible to imagine. As libertarians are the philosophical guardians of self-government, so libertines are the unethical apotheosis of misrule. Libertarians espouse self-government, libertines misrule. One is a moral and political ideal, the other an excuse for an abandonment of ideals.

This is related to a distinction drawn by Ronald Dworkin, that between Liberty as Licence and Liberty as Independence. It is necessary, Dworkin insists, to distinguish

---

[33] Savulescu and Persson, "Moral Enhancement, Freedom and the God Machine", <http://www.ncbi.nlm.nih.gov/pmc/articles/PMC3431130/pdf/ukmss-49380.pdf>, p. 13.
[34] <http://www.britannica.com/EBchecked/topic/385345/Lord-of-Misrule>.

between the idea of liberty as license, that is, the degree to which a person is free from social or legal constraint to do what he might wish to do, and liberty as independence, that is, the status of a person as independent and equal rather than subservient . . .

And it is independence which is at the heart of my opposition to moral enhancement of the sort espoused by Julian, Ingmar, and others. Dworkin continues:

> Liberty as license is an indiscriminate concept because it does not distinguish among forms of behaviour. Every prescriptive law diminishes liberty as license: good laws, like laws prohibiting murder, diminish this liberty in the same way, and possibly to a greater degree, as bad laws like laws prohibiting political speech. The question raised by any such law is not whether it attacks liberty, which it does, but whether the attack is justified by some competing value, like equality, or safety or public amenity. If a social philosopher places a very high value on liberty as license, he may be understood as arguing for a lower relative value for these competing values. If he defends freedom of speech, for example, by some general argument in favor of license, then his argument also supports, at least, pro tanto, freedom to form monopolies or smash storefront windows.
>
> But liberty as independence is not an indiscriminate concept in that way, it may well be, for example, that laws against murder or monopoly do not threaten but are necessary to protect, the political independence of citizens generally . . . If he argues for freedom of speech, for example, on some general argument in favor of independence and equality, he does not automatically argue in favor of greater license when these other values are not at stake.[35]

So Mill did not advocate the sort of freedom to do wrong which the law controls. But he recognized, as Julian and Ingmar do not, that the law is not infallible, and the room, the independence, it leaves citizens to form their own values and choose their own way of life is vital for a free society—a society in which even basic laws may be changed for compelling reasons. The God Machine takes away the independence of decision-making, of thought which can lead to action, this is why it is incompatible with both independence and autonomy, incompatible with both liberty as licence and liberty as independence. The God Machine, unlike Milton's God, is heavily into subservience and completely abolishes independence.

Here they are being (to put the point in the most charitable way possible) inconsistent. They have admitted that it will only appear to

---

[35] Ronald Dworkin, *Taking Rights Seriously* (London: Duckworth, 1977), pp. 262–3.

the agent that she has changed her mind, the God Machine will have changed it for her.

More important by far, Mill, when he talks of the exercise of power over others, is talking about legitimate power exercised through law or peer pressure, both of which leave the agent ultimately free to disagree and disobey and when enforced by law, leave open the possibility of law reform. In extreme cases Mill would also include harm used in self-defence or violence against assailants to prevent harm to third parties who can and often do fight back. But Mill imagines that the justification for the exercise of this power will be revealed by consideration of the merits of the case, as I have consistently argued, merits that are accessible to reason "all things considered".[36] Such "justifications" engineered without opportunity for either scrutiny, consideration, justification, or redress, out of sight and beyond mind, by a God Machine that is neither accountable nor indeed controllable constitute tyranny properly so-called.

The God Machine, if it knows what's good for it (and "by God!" it would know just that), would never allow itself to be switched off or disconnected and it would justify this decision to itself, following Persson and Savulescu, as being in humanity's own best interests.

The God Machine is after all how Persson and Savulescu themselves have made it, in their own image so to speak: "the most powerful, self-learning, self-developing bioquantum computer ever constructed".

John Stuart Mill of his own free will would never have put himself or anyone else in the power of such a beast. Following Mill, I stand by my own claims, in this book and elsewhere; that unlike Milton's God, Persson and Savulescu's God Machine and its equivalents are both unattractive as moral enhancers or if they are not strictly moral enhancers, unattractive as Gods; unlike Milton's version.[37]

---

[36] John Harris, "Taking Liberties with Free Fall", *Journal of Medical Ethics*, vol. 40, no. 6 (2014): 371–4; John Harris, "Moral Progress and Moral Enhancement", *Bioethics*, vol. 27, no. 5 (2013): 285–90; John Harris, "What It's Like to be Good", *Cambridge Quarterly of Healthcare Ethics*, vol. 21, no. 3 (2012): 293–305; John Harris, "'Ethics is for Bad Guys!': Putting the 'Moral' into Moral Enhancement", *Bioethics*, vol. 27, no. 3 (2013): 169–73; Chan and Harris, "Moral Enhancement and Prosocial Behaviour".

[37] This chapter was presented at the "Fellows Seminar" of The Centre for Advanced Study in Bioethics Westfälische Wilhelms-Universität, Münster. I am grateful to all the participants for helpful comments. A version appeared as John Harris, "How Narrow the Strait: The God Machine and the Spirit of Liberty", *Cambridge Quarterly of Healthcare Ethics*, vol. 23, no. 3 (2014): 247–60.

7

"Ethics is for Bad Guys!"
Putting the "Moral" into Moral Enhancement

7.1 The Moral of Moral Enhancement

To explore the limitations of moral bioenhancement further we can scarcely do better than consult our simian relatives who are also with us as representatives of our evolutionary past. In doing so we will be exploring the nature of ethics because of course we need to know what morality is in order to enhance it.

The famous three wise monkeys who appear in a seventeenth-century carving over a door of the famous Tōshō guō shrine in Nikkō Japan are represented covering their eyes, ears, and mouth and are "saying" so to speak, "see no evil, hear no evil, speak no evil". Sometimes in folklore a fourth monkey, perhaps a little wiser than the others, is depicted as saying "do no evil".

Tom Douglas has invited us to consider a further step, a step which I believe will be a step too far, namely altering the minds of monkeys and indeed humans so that they *cannot want to do evil*. There is a difference between deliberately averting one's gaze, or turning a blind eye, or stopping one's ears and deliberately making oneself blind, deaf, dumb, and cognitively impaired!

The poet, Adrian Mitchell, memorably adapted this parable in a polemical poem which he had conceived as an overt political act. He first recited his poem in public (I believe), "To Whom It May Concern (Tell Me Lies About Vietnam)", at a Vietnam war protest rally in Trafalgar Square, in 1964. I was there; listening, and protesting. Here is the refrain:

> So scrub my skin with women
> Chain my tongue with whisky

> Stuff my nose with garlic,
> Coat my eyes with butter
> Fill my ears with silver
> Stick my legs in plaster
> Tell me lies about Vietnam.[1]

Mitchell was, among many other things, pointing to strategies of oblivion which can help make the unacceptable palatable and pointing to the fact that you would have to be blind, deaf, dumb, and numbed in the ways he describes, not to cry out against the Vietnam war.

Douglas is, in a sense, recommending the opposite: strategies for making the unacceptable unpalatable. But Douglas goes further, he countenances making the unacceptable undoable!

Tom Douglas has suggested:

Suppose I believe that I ought to be more moved by the plight of the global poor, and ought to do more to help them. However, I have trouble drumming up much sympathy for them. To remedy this, I decide to dedicate half an hour every evening, for one month, to watching disturbing and graphic images of the effects of poverty. This is an attempt at moral enhancement via the direct modulation of emotions, without cognitive mediation. It seems to fall within the scope of Harris' critique. Yet it again it is not clear that my action here is morally impermissible or undesirable.

Thus, to the extent that Harris' concerns are meant to support a general indictment of emotional moral enhancement, they seem to be at odds with our intuitions about at least some cases.[2]

I should say again that, contra Douglas, I have no objection whatsoever to moral bioenhancement generally, nor to moral enhancement of the emotions in particular, nor do I, nor did I, wish to propose any "general indictment" of emotional moral enhancement. My concern is with the possibility of achieving such noble objectives in ways that would actually be enhancing, let alone morally enhancing, and without compromising our freedom. Now Douglas is also suggesting that if I do not object to emotional modulation of the practical kind, I should not, cannot consistently, find fault with more effective interventions, chemical, or possibly genetic.

---

[1] <http://www.bloodaxebooks.com/poemsample15.asp>, accessed 2 June 2011.
[2] Tom Douglas, "Moral Enhancement via Direct Emotion Modulation: A Reply to John Harris", *Bioethics*, vol. 27, no. 3 (2013): 160–8, at p. 163.

The problem with this approach is that moral emotions are not simply dual use but multi-purpose. Douglas again:

Of course, they may be motivated by reasoning, or other cognitive processes, but that is also true of paradigmatic examples of emotional moral enhancement: for example, the direct pharmaceutical modulation of emotion. The distinctive feature of emotional moral enhancement is that, once the enhancement has been initiated, there is no further need for cognition: emotions are modified directly. This appears to be the case with stimulus avoidance. However, stimulus avoidance can, intuitively, be morally permissible, and indeed morally desirable. Perhaps it would be better if the philanderer simply resisted his temptations to cheat, or used other, cognitive means of changing his behaviour. But assuming that all superior methods have been exhausted, stimulus avoidance seems to be a prima facie acceptable strategy.[3]

This is an interesting and revealing passage and one that goes to the heart of my disagreement with Douglas, and indeed to the core of my own approach to ethics. For over thirty years in my classes on moral philosophy I have emphasized to students who are inclined to rely on moral emotions: love, altruism, sympathy, and the like, that love is great for lovers and altruism and sympathy are good feelings to have. But what if they are not felt, or worse not felt for particular groups, racial, national, religious political; or for particular individuals? That is when you need moral philosophy, moral reasoning.

7.2 Ethics is for Bad Guys

Ethics is for bad guys! The good don't need ethics, but the truly good in this sense are so few and far between that few of us ever encounter them. Ethics is for those occasions on which compassion, altruism, and basic decency fail; or for those people who fail to think and feel for and about others given what will happen to others or to the world if they do not, or who are not disposed to do as they should! Moral reasoning is needed to identify the appropriate objects for sympathy, empathy, and the sort of generalized love, concern, respect, and protection that is the conclusion of a moral argument and which is often expressed as the so-called "golden rule"—"love thy neighbour as thyself". We will, I believe, always need to use moral reasoning to act as a guide to our emotions and as a

---

[3] Douglas, "Moral Enhancement via Direct Emotion Modulation", pp. 162–3.

way of checking that we are having appropriate feelings in appropriate circumstances and for appropriate objects.

If (though I doubt it) the good involves feeling the right way, how do we know that we are feeling the right way?

A moral agent, whatever else she may be, is someone who cares about doing the right thing, someone for whom the difference between right and wrong is important. Such a person will always want to ask him or herself if what feels right is right. And the answer to this question cannot be provided by a second consultation of one's feelings or worse by simply intuiting how one feels about things.

The history of ethics is in great part a history of the struggle to understand who and what are the appropriate objects of our moral concern and the reasons why such individuals matter and indeed what it is that makes it incumbent upon us to respect them in certain ways. The effect of this struggle has been consistently to deepen and refine the ambit of our moral concern; to, for example, embrace women and children equally, to extend our moral concern to other races, other nations, other religions, and, in contemporary debate, to consider appropriate ways to feel about and act towards humans at different stages of development: embryos or those in PVS for example or indeed to animals.

When someone says: "The distinctive feature of emotional moral enhancement is that, once the enhancement has been initiated, there is no further need for cognition: emotions are modified directly" alarm bells should ring. So long as we have rock solid guarantees that our directly modified emotions are of the right sort and will have the right effects all might be expected to be well. Since we know we cannot have such guarantees, we will never have "no further need for cognition". More, we know we must keep rationality at the centre of moral enhancement.

7.3 The Strategy of Avoiding Thought

Another philosopher, very different from Douglas, is also notorious for trying to do away with moral philosophy and rely directly on feelings. Leon Kass talking about cloning notoriously says:

We are repelled by the prospect of cloning human beings not because of the strangeness or novelty of the undertaking, but because we intuit and feel, immediately and without argument, the violation of things that we rightfully hold dear.[4]

I am surprised to find myself comparing Douglas and Kass, since Douglas is by far the more sophisticated philosopher. However, the difficulty that both share is of course, to know when one's sense of outrage, or one's "feelings" in Douglas's case, are evidence of something morally disturbing and when they are simply an expression of bare prejudice or simply an induced emotional response of the sort Douglas proposes. George Orwell[5] once memorably referred to this reliance on intuition or emotion as use of "moral nose"; as if one could simply sniff a situation and smell or feel the rightness or wrongness. The problem is that nasal reasoning is notoriously unreliable, and olfactory moral philosophy has done little to refine it or give it a respectable foundation. We should remember that in the recent past, among the many discreditable uses of so-called "moral feelings", people have been disgusted by the sight of Jews, black people, and indeed women being treated as equals and mixing on terms of equality with others. In the absence of convincing arguments, we should be suspicious of accepting the conclusions of those who use nasal reasoning or emotions as the basis of their moral convictions or indeed actions.

Kass disarmingly admits revulsion "is not an argument", but the problem is highlighted by his use of the term "rightfully".[6] How can we know that revulsion, however sincerely or vividly felt, is occasioned by the violation of things we rightfully hold dear unless we have a theory, or at least an argument, about which of the things we happen to hold dear or feel strongly about are things we *rightfully* hold dear? The term "rightfully" implies a judgement which confirms the respectability of the feelings. If it is simply one feeling confirming another, then we really

---

[4] Leon R. Kass, "The Wisdom of Repugnance", *The New Republic* (2 June 1997): 17–26.

[5] In a letter to Humphrey House, 11 April 1940: *The Collected Essays, Journalism and Letters of George Orwell*, vol. 1 (Harmondsworth: Penguin, 1970), p. 583. See my more detailed discussion of the problems with this type of reasoning in *Wonderwoman and Superman: The Ethics of Human Biotechnology* (Oxford: Oxford University Press, 1992), Chapter 2, and in my *Violence and Responsibility* (London: Routledge & Kegan Paul, 1980), p. 112. Orwell's idea has been taken up by others. See H. A. Chapman, D. A. Kim, J. M. Susskind, and A. K. Anderson, "In Bad Taste: Evidence for the Oral Origins of Moral Disgust", *Science*, vol. 323, no. 5918 (2009): 1222–6.

[6] Here the argument follows lines taken in John Harris, *Enhancing Evolution* (Princeton and Oxford: Princeton University Press, 2007), pp. 129ff.

are in the situation Wittgenstein lampooned as buying a second copy of the same newspaper to confirm the truth of what we read in the first.

7.4 The Avoidance of "Cognitive Mediation"

Think again of Douglas's example quoted earlier, in which Douglas imagines dedicating himself for "half an hour every evening, for one month, to watching disturbing and graphic images of the effects of poverty" to morally enhance himself. It is simply not true that the actions in this example are "without cognitive mediation" as Douglas claims. Douglas's strategy has been deliberately chosen and the reasons for the modulation of emotions involved are always available to and indeed present to the agent. It is hard to imagine that someone might forget why they have set themselves the grim task of watching "disturbing and graphic images". And again I agree with Douglas that his action in this case is neither "morally impermissible [nor] undesirable". I have never argued, nor never meant to imply, that moral enhancement generally or moral enhancement via inducing or exaggerating particular emotions is either impermissible or undesirable. I have simply expressed three sorts of scepticism or worry. One about the likelihood that so-called moral enhancement of the emotions would be likely to work, and secondly I have argued that insofar as it did work it would probably have a deleterious effect on freedom, and thirdly, as I have argued here, tinkering with the emotions is not a form of moral enhancement at all. It is more like the threat of punishment; it may make immoral behaviour less likely, but it does not enhance morality.[7]

In short, emotional moral enhancement is simply ethically otiose. Douglas knows what's right; he doesn't need moral enhancement to deliver his moral conclusions. If he believes he "ought to be more moved by the plight of the global poor" it is surely (hopefully?) for good reasons. These reasons do not include how he happens to feel, they are the reasons he has for wanting to feel in a particular way. These reasons necessarily have cognitive content. The feelings are posterior to

---

[7] John Harris and Sarah Chan, "Moral Behaviour is Not What It Seems", *Proceedings of the National Academy of Sciences USA*, Early Edition (2010): <http://www.pnas.org/cgi/doi/10.1073/pnas.1015001107>; Sarah Chan and John Harris, "Moral Enhancement and Prosocial Behaviour", *Journal of Medical Ethics*, vol. 37, no. 3 (2011): 130–1.

the reasons—if he didn't have the reasons he would not search for the feelings. What is doubtful is that this process works the other way. Do we start with the feelings and then try to work out why they are appropriate? I have to admit that we sometimes do and we sometimes find our feelings are inappropriate or misplaced. The crucial question is not which way round the process occurs but whether it is feelings or thought that are the more reliable?

Is the drummed-up sympathy supposed to confirm his clearly appropriate judgements about what the global poor need? Clearly not! Douglas knows what's right and needs no moral enhancement, for these purposes at least. He may need some help in feeling sympathy but that is a different problem and not, I would suggest, a moral one. I don't feel sympathy for many of the people who need my help. The needy can, after all, be a repulsive lot! That perhaps is part of their tragedy (or part of mine). The sympathy is not the cause of my understanding that the poor need help. Rather it is my understanding that the poor need and deserve help that is the occasion of my sympathy. Sympathy is not a brute emotion or feeling, it is not a visceral reaction, something that wells up within us and needs explanation. The moral sympathy is occasioned by understanding, an understanding of the plight, the situation of the poor. It is occasioned by an understanding of their needs and what they will suffer if those needs are not met. I don't have to be nice to be good. This perhaps is part of what I take to be Douglas's mistake. I just have to know what's right and to know that I ought to do what's right. Where there is weakness of will (akrasia), the problem is not one that requires moral enhancement but something akin to "stiffening the sinews" and "summoning up the blood".

Douglas's problem seems to me to be that he equates moral enhancement with having the right feelings. Socrates was surely close when he saw it as a combination of knowing the good and doing the good. If and when there is a gulf between these two there may be no reliable way of filling it. Weakness of will seems to be a perennial problem but it is not the same as absence of moral emotions and no one has yet shown that emotional enhancement has any greater likelihood of bridging the gap between thought and action than anything else. Feeling the good is no closer to doing the good than is knowing the good. And it suffers from the distinct disadvantage that, lacking cognitive content, feeling the good is indistinguishable from feeling the bad—except by an analysis of what will follow all things considered.

All moral philosophers, and indeed all ethicists, must have an interest in moral enhancement. I certainly do. To date the best, the most promising methods we have of moral enhancement are firstly I believe the traditional ones: education, parental and peer group guidance, social and personal example, and indeed reflection on what's right, namely ethics which is, properly understood, the science of the good. Recently, methods of cognitive enhancement have emerged which also show promise as moral enhancers and I have also endorsed these elsewhere.[8] We may hope to discover new and even more effective methods and I am not at all averse to the attempt made by Douglas and others so to do. For the moment, however, I have some reservations both about their likely success and as to whether they actually do constitute moral enhancement. It seems to me that moral enhancement properly so called must not only make the doing of good or right actions more probable and the doing of bad ones less likely, but must also include the understanding of what constitutes right and wrong action.

As I have suggested earlier in this book, there is no virtue in doing what you must.[9] If, as Douglas insists, "once the enhancement has been initiated, there is no further need for cognition", then the morally enhanced action is effectively automatic, unconscious, and therefore unintended, entirely outside the realm of moral responsibility and probably of criminal responsibility also. And of course the consequences for criminal responsibility of direct emotional interventions which bypass cognition, will need considerable further attention, particularly as and when other interventions to produce so-called "pro-social behaviour" take hold.[10]

Just as I may not be held responsible in any sense for behaviour which is quite literally outside my control, I also cannot be described as acting morally or virtuously if I behave automatically (unless I have declined to

---

[8] In Harris, *Enhancing Evolution*, Chapter 3, and Henry Greely, Barbara Sahakian, John Harris, Ron Kessler, Michael Gazzaniga, Philip Campbell, and Martha Farah, "Towards Responsible Use of Cognitive Enhancing Drugs by the Healthy", *Nature*, vol. 456, no. 7223 (2008): 702–5.

[9] John Harris, "Moral Enhancement and Freedom", *Bioethics*, vol. 25, no. 2 (2011): 102–11.

[10] Molly J. Crockett, Luke Clark, Marc D. Hauser, and Trevor W. Robbins, "Serotonin Selectively Influences Moral Judgment and Behavior through Effects on Harm Aversion", *Proceedings of the National Academy of Sciences USA*, vol. 107, no. 40 (2010): 17433–8. See also Chan and Harris, "Moral Enhancement and Prosocial Behaviour".

exercise cognitive control over automatic behaviour). Actions that are not under voluntary control, are not mine in any real sense at all. Of course there are things that I might find myself doing or find out that I have done, that I consciously adopt retrospectively but then of course they become the subject of further cognition and are self-consciously "made my own".

I simply do not see how movements (we cannot call them actions) whether virtuous or vicious in effect, can be part of the doings of a moral agent and therefore can constitute the morally enhanced doings of such an agent. Douglas and other proponents of forms of emotional moral enhancement which are beyond the reach of cognition and hence of intentional action are not functioning in the realm of morality.

7.5 Socrates' Conclusion is Also Mine

When, in *The Apology*,[11] Socrates famously explains to his accusers why he had devoted his life to criticism of others and of the state, he self-consciously sums up his life and identifies his life's work. He remarks that the important thing is to consider only whether in doing anything one is doing right or wrong, acting the part of a good man or a bad, and when Socrates concludes that "the greatest good of man is daily to converse about virtue...and that the life which is unexamined is not worth living", he sets out what might be considered the minimum conditions for moral agency and hence the conditions also for the rational attempt to lead a good life. Of course this is not the only defensible view about what moral agency might consist in. However I cling, perhaps dysfunctionally, to the view that moral enhancement worthy of the name needs to maintain its connection with the attempt to lead a good life oneself, and to help other moral agents to do the same.

So far from methods of moral enhancement which have "no further need for cognition" and in which "emotions are modified directly", I believe strongly (and hope that here and elsewhere I have given strong reasons for believing) that morality necessarily involves the self-conscious

---

[11] Plato, *The Apology*, trans. Benjamin Jowett: <http://classics.mit.edu//Plato/apology.html>. I use the Internet version since I am writing this in Italy, far from the four volumes of my own much-loved Jowett translation of Plato (but a little nearer geographically and spiritually to the scene of the trial of Socrates).

examination of one's actions and indeed one's life. Only self-conscious reflection on conduct can deliver answers to the question as to whether what one feels is right is indeed right. It is only such an examination, and the resolve to put its conclusions into effect, that constitute a moral life and, *a fortiori*, a morally enhanced life.[12]

[12] I wish to thank Sarah Chan for helpful comments.

8

Molecules and Morality

Tell me where is fancy bred,
Or in the heart or in the head?
How begot, how nourished?
ALL: Reply, Reply.
It is engendered in the eyes,
With gazing fed, and Fancy dies
In the cradle where it lies;
Let us all ring Fancy's knell.
I'll begin it. Ding, dong, bell . . . [1]

This song, from Shakespeare's *The Merchant of Venice*, is sung while Bassanio chooses the casket which could give him his (and Portia's) heart's desire or will blight his and her life forever. The lesson is that while fancy (a cross between desire and appreciation) may be engendered in the eyes, it dies quickly. What is needed is not fancy, but judgement; and that is what Bassanio relies on in making his choice. Indeed *The Merchant of Venice* is a play all about judgement and misjudgement. Too often, in contemporary neuroscience, judgement is banished altogether and with it reasoning as a spur for conduct or conclusions is also banished. So let us all ring fancy's knell . . .

A different account, and one that we shall re-examine now, tells us that fancy, and indeed true love and true morality, are neither bred in the heart nor in the head, at least as Shakespeare understood these ideas, but are the results of molecules acting on the brain.[2]

---

[1] William Shakespeare, *The Merchant of Venice*, Act 3, Scene 2. The Arden Shakespeare, *Complete Works*, ed. Richard Proudfoot, Ann Thomson, and David Scott Kastan (Walton-on-Thames: Thomas Nelson and Sons, 1998), p. 844.

[2] Hormones are compounds produced by an endocrine gland and released into the bloodstream. A neurotransmitter on the other hand is a compound released from a nerve terminal. Some molecules are both hormones and neurotransmitters, depending on the

Neuroscience, as we have noted, is now developing interventions that act directly on the brain influencing behaviour, attitudes, and dispositions, affecting motivation, and, some claim, raising the possibility of adding moral enhancement to physical and cognitive enhancement. These possibilities, if that is what they are, raise important issues of liberty and responsibility which not only affect our sense of who and of what we are, but literally of the extent to which we are, or can remain, masters of our fate, entities which create ourselves by our decisions and actions.

A recent report of the Royal Society, of which I was a co-author, put it thus:

> The human brain is not viewed in the same way as other organs. The brain holds the key to mind and behaviour, and so to most it has a 'special' status. The relatively young field of neuroscience is the study of the brain and nervous system. The law is concerned with regulating behaviour, and so it is reasonable to ask whether and if so how neuroscience could or should inform the law.[3]

In addition of course to the interest of the law in criminal and moral responsibility and in what the brain might tell us about past, and predictable future, actions, we all have an interest both for ourselves and others in the way in which our and their behaviour and dispositions to act might be influenced for better or worse. In short how moral enhancement and its opposite might be able to affect our present and future behaviour and indeed our access to memory of past behaviour or our ability to manipulate those memories in various ways.

8.1 Is There a Science of Morality?

As I have said, "how to be good?" is the pre-eminent question for ethics, although one that philosophers and ethicists seldom address head on.

Knowing how to be good, or perhaps more modestly and more accurately, knowing how to go about trying to be good, is of immense theoretical and practical importance. This "know how" is the business of

mode of release—so essentially the difference between hormones and neurotransmitters is semantic.

[3] The Royal Society, *Brain Waves Module 4: Neuroscience and the Law*. ISBN: 978-0-85403-932-6, December 2011, p. iii. See also *Brain Waves Module 1*. ISBN: 978-0-85403-879-4.

a science of the good. It is also perhaps the most important issue facing contemporary neuroscience, social policy, and criminal justice. The links between this highly theoretical question and the preoccupations of contemporary neuroscience and the interests of the criminal law and indeed of those preoccupied with social policy, education, and the common good will be explored in this presentation. They are examined, however, through a lens which focuses on debates about how to effect moral enhancement or moral improvement in human beings.

If, for example, the Human Brain Project[4] relies on data interpreted according to theories such as the ones we are about to examine, it will make some very fundamental mistakes of understanding. Particularly, if the neuroscience of morality is misconceived, then any "data" produced and recorded will not help our understanding very much. So I want now to examine one very particular group of possible sources of error.

In a recent book, *Braintrust*, Patricia Smith Churchland[5] sums up a long career spent trying to persuade us that the mind is the brain and all the men and women merely . . . if not neurones, at least machines in the ghost. Indeed Churchland has a somewhat unique status in the philosophy of neuroscience. Although she does pretty much think we are indeed just neurones: "What", she asks, "does it mean for a system of neurones to care about or value something?"[6] The answer of course is that neurones do not have a care in the world. The tale Churchland tells is one expressing a particular materialist theory of the mind and one that fits with a set of such theories which may or may not be sustainable, depending on how they are interpreted. What she also defends is, I believe, a demonstrably erroneous theory of morality.

Let's start with what Churchland has got absolutely right . . . and it is a very great deal. She says quite rightly, and repeats . . . repeatedly, that morality is "tethered to . . . has its foundations on . . . is constrained by . . . anchored to . . . prefigured in . . . " our evolutionary origins.[7] She calls this being "tethered to the 'hard and fast'".[8] This is transparently, but

---

[4] <https://www.humanbrainproject.eu/en_GB>.

[5] Patricia S. Churchland, *Braintrust: What Neuroscience Tells Us about Morality* (Princeton and Oxford: Princeton University Press, 2011). I am grateful to Raymond Tallis, Sarah Chan, Sadie Regmi, and Walter Glannon for helpful comments and suggestions in the remainder of this chapter.

[6] Churchland, *Braintrust*, p. 1.   [7] Churchland, *Braintrust*, pp. 1–18.

[8] Churchland, *Braintrust*, p. 2.

trivially, correct; so long, that is, as one takes a not very rigorous view of what terms like "constrained" or "tethered" mean. Indeed, this could be said more or less plausibly of almost any contemporary feature of humans and indeed of slugs and snails and puppy dogs' tails. How are we tethered to our evolutionary past—as apes or as their mono-cellular forebears?

Having thus purported to establish firm foundations, Churchland goes on to build an edifice that moves seamlessly from the hard and fast to the fast and loose.[9]

What Churchland does not talk about, but seems to assume, is just how constraining these constraints on what morality might be like are.[10] Having attempted to sell us on the idea of firm foundations (and who would be rash enough to reject these?) Churchland seems to think she has liberty and licence to make claims that, while consistent with such foundations, are no more entailed by them than, say, contemporary human thought is constrained by or tethered to, whatever arbitrary stage of the evolutionary antecedents of the human brain may be picked out for dramatic effect.

I suggest, (and have consistently argued), that what matters morally (and for that matter cognitively) is not where we come from but where we are, and where we are going. And our evolutionary past does not constrain or tether, but rather partially explains and indeed enables further development. Moreover, our evolutionary past does not predict in any material way and certainly does not significantly determine our future trajectory. To make sense of such an idea it would first be necessary to identify an instance, a slice, of that evolutionary past and explain the nature of that constraint. One such instance would have certainly been a mono-cellular organism, another our ape ancestor somewhere between 5 and 7 million years ago in Africa. I have argued that even now neither my, nor Churchland's, "nature" constrains to any significant extent (although it may explain features of) our evolutionary successors.[11]

---

[9] Students of the English language will note that I have moved here, for tendentious effect, between two different senses of what it is to be "fast" to different concepts which happen to be homophones.

[10] Raymond Tallis, *Aping Mankind* (Durham: Acumen, 2011), Chapters 3 and 8.

[11] John Harris, *Wonderwoman and Superman: The Ethics of Human Biotechnology* (Oxford: Oxford University Press, 1992), and John Harris, *Enhancing Evolution* (Princeton and Oxford: Princeton University Press, 2007).

I appreciate that we humans and our successors, are likely to remain organic (or partially organic) and carbon based, but those "constraints" are not germane here. It is salutary to be sure, to remind ourselves of our evolutionary past, our humble origins if you like; there are lessons to be learned; but we are no more constrained by our ape ancestry than apes were by their slug (or equivalent) ancestry and so ad infinitum. Just as human imagination and human thought is not constrained by simian imagination and thought, still less by sluggish imagination and thought, human morality is equally "free".[12]

So let's look at what Churchland makes of her freedom. She draws very pessimistic conclusions from the fact that there are moral disagreements. Let's look at one of the moral dilemmas of which she does attempt a lengthy analysis.

Within our own culture there is often disagreement about the evaluation of an act. In 1972 bush pilot Martin Hartwell, courageously agreeing to fly a mercy flight despite bad weather, tragically crashed the bush plane. His passengers included an Inuit child who desperately needed an appendectomy and a nurse along to care for him. The nurse died on impact, and eventually the child died as well. With two broken legs, starving and near death after many weeks of waiting in vain for rescue, Hartwell consumed the leg of his friend, the dead nurse. Eventually after 31 days in the bitter cold, Hartwell was rescued. On cannibalism in such extreme circumstances, opinion varies greatly, and I am doubtful that there is a uniquely correct answer, even when all the details of the story are known. Many well-fed people are horrified at the prospect of eating their dog, but the traditional Inuit are comparably horrified at the idiocy of starving to death when eating a dog would keep life going until game was found. As we all know well, rational people may disagree about the best way to handle taxation, or education of the young, or when to wage pre-emptive wars. Often there are better or worse choices, but no uniquely right choice; in such cases, constraint satisfaction does its business-balancing and harmonizing and settling on a suitable decision.[13]

Churchland's analysis of this case is worrying and reveals severe limitations to her approach to ethics, seeing it, as she does, not as simply based on, but consisting entirely of, emotional reactions tethered to and arising from the putative evolutionary origins of morality. I say "putative" because as I have argued at length elsewhere,[14] morality is more

---

[12] Harris, *Enhancing Evolution*.   [13] Churchland, *Braintrust*, p. 25.
[14] John Harris, *The Value of Life* (London: Routledge, 1985); John Harris, *On Cloning* (London: Routledge, 2004); Harris, *Enhancing Evolution*.

appropriately judged of than felt,[15] and hence it is to rationality and its evolutionary origins, rather than to the emotions that we should look. And indeed, as we shall see, Churchland partially understands this. What is truly shocking, to adapt a famous remark of Ronald Dworkin, is not the idea that the evolutionary origins of morality count but of what counts as the evolutionary origins of morality.[16]

First another point of agreement. When Churchland says "I am doubtful that there is a uniquely correct answer . . . Often there are better or worse choices, but no uniquely right choice" she is saying something uncontroversial in a very large number of cases. There are sometimes uniquely correct answers, but even an objective theory of ethics does not have to accept this. What ethics is about is the morally best choice "all things considered".[17] But this is not how she analyses her case. What she argues is: "Many well-fed people are horrified at the prospect of eating their dog, but the traditional Inuit are comparably horrified at the idiocy of starving to death when eating a dog would keep life going until game was found." What we are asked to compare is two opposing but comparable emotional reactions; one group is "horrified" at one thing, others at another. Since the horror, I assume, is assumed to be equal (comparable but un-measurable) there is we are asked to believe no basis for rational choice. If morality consists of attitudes or emotions, if it consists of feelings, then the only way in is via either the strength of the feelings or their sincerity. Since there is not much prospect of an independent measure of either of these we are left to take the protagonists' word for it.

And this is a big problem. If "there are better or worse choices", what makes them better or worse? It can't be simply how we feel about them, for then the only way of answering the perfectly reasonable question as to why we believe what we affect to be horrified by, is really horrifying, worthy of being horrified by, is to feel what we feel all over again. Why, in short, is what we are actually horrified by the sort of thing that it is appropriate or reasonable to be horrified by? If the answer is that we simply feel it so to be, then the only way of confirming the veracity or

---

[15] Contra some interpretations of David Hume, *A Treatise on Human Nature* (1738). This edition: London and New York: Everyman's Library, Dent and Dutton, 1966. Vol. II. Part One, p. 178.

[16] Ronald Dworkin, *Taking Rights Seriously* (London: Duckworth, 1977), p. 255.

[17] John Harris, "What It's Like to be Good", *Cambridge Quarterly of Healthcare Ethics*, vol. 21, no. 3 (2012): 293–305.

appropriateness of our response would be to contemplate the problem again and see if we still feel the same. And this leads to a familiar problem of circularity, as I have argued elsewhere:[18]

> If it is simply one feeling confirming another, then we really are in the situation Wittgenstein lampooned as buying a second copy of the same newspaper to confirm the truth of what we read in the first.[19] As Wittgenstein, albeit emphasising the obvious, insisted: "justification consists in appealing to something independent".[20]

It also cannot be that this independent arbiter of the morally better or worse choice is "constraint satisfaction . . . balancing and harmonizing and settling on a suitable decision" for it has to be a suitably *better* decision, and that means *morally* better, better from the perspective of some relevant ethical features.

I have written about the nature of morally relevant features extensively over the years[21] and indeed in Chapters 1 and 2 of this book. They are not esoteric; they are the things that make life go well or ill for people, that secure justice and protect rights and interests and secure liberty and autonomy. They have to do with harm and benefit, with health and sickness, safety and danger. They are good health as opposed to illness and injury, longer rather than shorter life, happiness rather than misery, pleasure not pain, good friends rather than bad enemies[22] and so almost ad infinitum. If you ask anyone to start a list of such things in rank order of importance the convergence would expectably be strong over the top half of the list with divergence increasing as desperation, or acute failure of the imagination, sets in. We all know what's good for us and even more clearly what isn't. Sometimes we are in doubt, and we can be wrong, but not enough to make prudence an illusion or benevolence incoherent.

---

[18] Harris, "What It's Like to be Good".

[19] Ludwig Wittgenstein, *Philosophical Investigations*, trans. G. E. M. Anscombe, 3rd edn. (Oxford: Basil Blackwell, 2001), para. 265, p. 79e.

[20] Wittgenstein, *Philosophical Investigations*, para. 265, p. 79e.

[21] See for example Harris, *The Value of Life*; Harris, *Enhancing Evolution*, Chapters 3, 4, and 6; John Harris, "The Concept of the Person and the Value of Life", *Kennedy Institute of Ethics Journal*, vol. 9, no. 4 (1999): 293–308.

[22] William Shakespeare, *Richard III*, Act 4, Scene 2. The Arden Shakespeare, p. 727.
KING RICHARD: Dar'st thou resolve to kill a friend of mine?
TYRELL: Please you; but I would rather kill two enemies.

If we are curious about what makes a choice best among all other possibilities, about what are the criteria of "bestness", it will be the one that, *inter alia*, best promotes justice, the rights and interests of persons, animals, and the planet and which best protects sentient individuals from suffering and harm.

We have seen that whatever these morally relevant features are they cannot be emotions like feeling horrified or disgusted or sickened by something or someone. These feelings are notoriously unreliable and susceptible to manipulation and prejudice of all sorts. They might of course be pro-social emotions, but that raises the underlying question what makes an emotion pro-social and a bigger question still: might there be a more pro-social but not emotionally stimulated alternative that is even better, in that it is even more pro-social?

The concept of pro-sociality can be analysed like any other concept. It has cognitive, not simply, or probably even, emotional content let alone molecular content. A pro-social emotion or a pro-social anything else is one that is literally "in favour of" or for the benefit of (pro) people or a society of people. Insofar as pro-sociality is a surrogate for, or equivalent of, morality it has to be plausibly related to good and bad, right and wrong. What such pro-social or moral "things" are, is a matter of evidence and argument, it is a matter of demonstrating in what ways action, policy, or emotion X is good for people or society.

8.2 Rationality not Emotionality

If we are to look for plausible evolutionary precursors of morality, rather than simply of cooperation, then rationality is a better bet than pro-sociality.[23] I put it no higher than this because frankly it doesn't matter what are the precursors, foundations, or roots of morality or the posts to which scapegoats are "tethered". What matters is what morality requires, not what proto-morality might have required long before Raquel Welch was fighting dinosaurs, and at a time when no one could even use language anyway! In those halcyon days, if anyone could have put the point, they might have just managed the great leap of intelligence performed by Churchland, namely to think that to let people die (assuming that they valued them) rather than eat a dog, was well, "idiocy"!

---

[23] Harris, "What It's Like to be Good".

Idiocy is in fact a great moral concept, and one aptly used more than once by Churchland.[24] The charge of "idiocy" implicitly relies upon the famous, both logical and ethical, device of drawing attention to the fact that certain beliefs, positions, rules, stances, etc. might simply be idiotic because they are self-defeating in terms of the agreed moral objectives: in this case saving the sorts of lives agreed to matter. Now self-defeating actions or policies are not necessarily pro-social in Churchland's (or Crockett's)[25] sense, even when they save lives, because Churchland is only interested in those lives whose mournful eyes (homage to Joan Baez)[26] are capable of engaging with those of the putative moral agent.

Churchland, in Chapter 7 of her book,[27] specifically repudiates maximizing the number of lives saved and hence repudiates all those mournful eyes which are beyond the narrow purview of her philosophy[28] or moral gaze; thereby aligning herself with the "innumerate" ethicists rightly ridiculed by Derek Parfit.[29] It is genuinely "stupid" to value lives, but only lives of those who can arouse our pity directly and emotionally, rather than also those lives which engage our moral concern, intellectually. If lives matter, then each life matters. As Jeremy Bentham famously said, each is to count for one and none for more than one.[30] And if one counts for one then two count for two; we thus need to be able to count as well as to feel. And even a morality

---

[24] Churchland, *Braintrust*, p. 5. Here the word she uses is "stupid".

[25] Molly J. Crockett, Luke Clark, Marc D. Hauser, and Trevor W. Robbins, "Serotonin Selectively Influences Moral Judgment and Behavior through Effects on Harm Aversion", *Proceedings of the National Academy of Sciences USA*, vol. 107, no. 40 (2010): 17433–8. See also John Harris and Sarah Chan, "Moral Behaviour is Not What It Seems", *Proceedings of the National Academy of Sciences USA*, Early Edition (2010): <http://www.pnas.org/cgi/doi/10.1073/pnas.1015001107>; Sarah Chan and John Harris, "Moral Enhancement and Prosocial Behaviour", *Journal of Medical Ethics*, vol. 37, no. 3 (2011): 130–1.

[26] <http://www.metrolyrics.com/donna-donna-lyrics-joan-baez.html>, accessed 2 March 2012.

[27] Churchland, *Braintrust*, p. 176.

[28] "There are more things in heaven and earth, Horatio, Than are dreamt of in your philosophy" (William Shakespeare, *Hamlet*, Act 1, Scene 5, lines 174–5. The Arden Shakespeare).

[29] Derek Parfit, "Innumerate Ethics", *Philosophy & Public Affairs*, vol. 7, no. 4 (1978): 285–301.

[30] Bentham's words are available to us only via John Stuart Mill's *Utilitarianism*, in this case in Mary Warnock's edition (London: Collins Fontana, 1962). Mill refers to "Bentham's dictum, 'everybody to count for one, nobody for more than one'" (Chapter V, p. 319).

remorselessly tethered to "the hard and fast" must recognize the hardness and fastness of basic numeracy.

As noted in the previous chapter: Ethics is for bad guys.[31] Ethics is for those occasions on which altruism, sympathy, and sociality fail; or for those people who fail to think and feel, or who are not disposed to do, as they should! It doesn't matter why ethics fails; it might fail for want of sympathy, or imagination, or serotonin or oxytocin; or it might fail to do right from weakness of will, or because those who need our concern, respect, and protection are out of sight. Moral reasoning is needed to identify the appropriate objects for sympathy, empathy, and the sort of generalized love, or at least concern, that is the conclusion of a moral argument and which is often expressed as "love thy neighbour as thyself".

Even English law, not the most progressive of vehicles for morality, recognizes that the idea of "neighbour" refers to more than vicinity. It is difficult to improve upon Lord Atkin's famous judgment in the seminal case of *Donoghue* v. *Stevenson*:[32]

Who then in law is my neighbour? The answer seems to be persons who are so closely and directly affected by my act that I ought reasonably to have them in contemplation as being so affected when I am directing my mind to the acts or omissions which are called in question.

It is reason that alerts us to what might be beyond our moral gaze and require our concern and which helps us to understand what we can and should do about it. We will, I believe, always need to use moral reasoning to act as a guide to our emotions and as a way of checking that we are having appropriate feelings in appropriate circumstances and for appropriate objects.

Pro-sociality is, as already noted, an idea, it is a concept, it has cognitive content and the behavioural expressions of that idea have consequences which make them plausible as expressions of that idea. Such consequences may also be inconsistent with or incommensurable with the idea, they may frustrate or even negate it.

Whatever the causal antecedents of pro-social behaviour are at the level of molecules, neuro-transmitters, or chemical compounds, if the

---

[31] John Harris, " 'Ethics is for Bad Guys!': Putting the 'Moral' into Moral Enhancement", *Bioethics*, vol. 27, no. 3 (2013): 169–73.

[32] *Donoghue* v. *Stevenson* [1932] UKHL 100 (26 May 1932).

behaviour is not, or if it ceases to be, intelligible as pro-social behaviour, then it simply isn't behaviour of that sort. A soul whose intentions are good is fated to be always misunderstood; if that is, those intentions do not do good at least a reasonable proportion of the time.

Pro-sociality, as is obvious and already indicated, has to be *pro*-social, it has to be in favour of or beneficial to, those people who are part of the polis, the relevant social group and pro-sociality, properly so called, has to have reasons as to why it is members of that group that are morally relevant.

And this is not a matter of intention, but of logic, or at least of argument. One such style of argument, per genus et differentiam, might show a coherent and defensible way of drawing the distinction between those who dwell within the "Pale" of moral concern and those who do not. "The Pale" from the early medieval period was the part of Ireland under the control of the "civilized" English. To dwell "beyond the Pale" was to be outside civilization and hence outside the scope of pro-social feelings.

At a time at which, as it is believed, pro-sociality was a mechanism for the protection of an in-group from aliens or outsiders, pro-sociality had no more connection with morality, than slugs have with humans. At such a stage in our evolutionary past, pro-sociality was *prudential*, not moral; or to use a less intentional and more objectively descriptive term, was *adaptive* rather than moral. We rightly distinguish acting out of self-interest, acting prudentially, from acting morally, in the interests of relevant others or the general good. It is only when adaptive mechanisms become understood by their users to the point when the purposes they serve are understood and the underlying rationale can be generalized for a reason, to all relevant cases, do they become moral. Of course self-defence against strangers who threaten our lives is usually moral, but not because they are aliens but because they are murderous.

Moreover, behaviour that is simply prudential will only be pro-social if it operates in the interests of relevant others. Our distant ancestors who favoured "their own kind" and cared nothing for aliens or outsiders, are no more acting morally than those who today favour their own kind in a way that does not relevantly in moral (not merely prudential) terms, distinguish their own kind from other kinds. The history of our species is tragically replete with people who believed it right to favour their own kind, defined in gender, racial, religious, or nationalistic terms. Killing those who were not members of the relevant in-group was never pro-social if it was done for that reason alone.

And it is human imagination that is one of the most potent of cognitive faculties that enables us to put ourselves into, if not the shoes of relevant others, at least into an understanding of the nature and consequences of our acts and decisions, and of the effects of those decisions on others and the world. The answer to a "what if . . . " question is not just a series of facts or propositions, it involves a set of imaginative understandings. To be sure some of this involves understanding "what it would feel like if . . . " but this is not what Churchland has in mind. She is equivocal over consequences, approving of Mill's utilitarianism for the importance it accords to happiness, yet on the same page rejects any imperative to maximize happiness.[33]

Without any sense of irony or inconsistency she admires Mill for his identifying that the "moral sphere is fundamentally about conduct that injures, damages or harms others or their interests"[34] but again shows herself to be morally innumerate,[35] by apparently also holding that this gives us no reason to minimize the perpetration of such harms, execrating those she calls "maximising consequentialists"[36] for wanting to minimize such harms and therefore maximize the benefits of accepting consequentialism. It is difficult to know how to take seriously someone who professes to believe in a morality that tries to minimize harms "to others or their interest" but sees no imperative to minimize the numbers of such others who are adversely affected by such harms and hence maximize the good that such a morality can deliver.

Churchland, like many others, misunderstands Bentham's famous injunction that each is to count for one and none for more than one, and that equality means "equal consideration for all"[37] to imply that we must always favour strangers over our own children when there are more of them or when favouring strangers does more good.

The idea that all persons are equal and that each counts the same is a political principle. It speaks to treatment sanctioned by laws, officials, and institutions. Equality and numerate ethics do not require that mothers must sometimes abandon their own children in favour of the children of others, and all but the most unreflective consequentialists know this. This does not of course imply that mothers must never put the

---

[33] Churchland, *Braintrust*, p. 177.   [34] Churchland, *Braintrust*, p. 177.
[35] Parfit, "Innumerate Ethics".   [36] Churchland, *Braintrust*, p. 178.
[37] Churchland, *Braintrust*, p. 178.

interests of others before those of their children, nor that they and theirs should make no sacrifices to secure benefits for others. It means that such sacrifices must be proportionate[38] and of course Churchland is not unaware of the importance of proportionality. However the law must treat all as equals, and so must governments and officials charged with distributing public goods, keeping the peace, and preserving the public health.[39] I talk of treatment "as equals" rather than of "equal treatment" following the distinction made famous by Ronald Dworkin,[40] who also incidentally explained how maximizing principles could be used according to this principle to justify treating two of one's own children "as equals" but unequally.

There is no sense in which moral judgement, properly so called[41] (moral thinking rather than moral feeling), is less "tethered to the hard and fast" or less rooted in our evolutionary origins than is serotonin, or oxytocin-induced "touchy-feely" responses. Churchland's own methodology does not require this, I believe, narrow conception of the lessons to be learned from evolution, nor from modern neuroscience. Each of these teaches us that cognition (thinking and judgement) is better, morally, intellectually, in terms of reliability and in terms of suiting means to ends, than is primitive pro-sociality—pro-sociality which relies on molecular or chemical stimuli unmediated by reason. Any successful science of the good will be based on, and dare I say "tethered to" judgement not feelings.

---

[38] The calculation of proportionality is not easy but it is certainly something for which rationality rather than emotions is required.

[39] John Coggon, *What Makes Health Public? A Critical Evaluation of Moral, Legal, and Political Claims in Public Health* (Cambridge: Cambridge University Press, 2012).

[40] Dworkin, *Taking Rights Seriously*, pp. 227 ff.

[41] Harris, "What It's Like to be Good".

9

Moral Progress and Moral Enhancement

This book, as well as developing a thesis about the nature of morality, its objectivity and potential enhancement also constitutes, as will already be obvious, an ongoing debate with other scholars about these issues. Prominent among these scholars are Ingmar Persson and Julian Savulescu who have thoughtfully reminded me that "because humans now have at their disposal technology so powerful that it could bring about the destruction of the whole planet if misused"[1] it is a seriously important matter that this misuse does not occur.

I have been actively campaigning against this misuse since I joined the Campaign for Nuclear Disarmament (CND) and took part in the Aldermaston Marches[2] in the UK from around 1960. This, almost lifelong, interest in the use and abuse of technology perhaps explains a certain obsessiveness in my theoretical interest in these issues.

I would like briefly to correct a few misunderstandings that have occurred in the lively debate between Persson, Savulescu, and I, misunderstandings that have arisen over the uses and abuses of moral enhancement as one technique or strategy for averting disaster.

In a recent contribution to this debate[3] Persson and Savulescu (P&S) spend a great deal of energy trying to support their claim that doing harm is both easier than preventing harm and also easier than doing good to the same degree. I had disagreed with them about this more out of a cussed belief that this claim was obviously wrong than because it was

---

[1] Ingmar Persson and Julian Savulescu, "Getting Moral Enhancement Right: The Desirability of Moral Bioenhancement", *Bioethics*, vol. 27, no. 3 (2013): 124–31. In response to John Harris, "Moral Enhancement and Freedom", *Bioethics*, vol. 25, no. 2 (2011): 102–11.

[2] And the less noticed "High Wycombe March".

[3] Persson and Savulescu, "Getting Moral Enhancement Right".

particularly crucial to the issue of moral enhancement. However, although I believe that doing harm and preventing harm are not in principle necessarily easier the one than the other, of course there are many particular cases where the balance will be skewed in a particular direction. In their attempted rebuttal of my claim that both these modalities, doing good and preventing harm, are both essential and equally effective ways of making the world a better and a safer place, they don't seem to me to have done much but show that one can indeed easily do a lot of good, and yes, one can indeed easily do a lot of harm. However, the issue only matters if there is some reason why we cannot both try to prevent harm and at the same time do good; so in a real sense this part of our disagreement is strictly "academic". However, this does not mean that it is not worth showing that this particular debate while interesting is yet another cog that is not connected to the machinery and though it certainly turns nothing turns with it.

9.1 Taking One's Chances

Before turning briefly to some of the issues that are still live it is worth noting an odd dissonance in P&S's way of taking about opportunities for good and evil. They start by noting that:

most readers of this paper probably have access to a car and live in densely populated areas. Whenever you drive, you could easily kill a number of people by ploughing into a crowd. But, we dare say, very few of you have the opportunity every day to save an equal number of lives.

They then go on to point out that:

It might be thought that our claim is undermined by the fact that we in affluent countries could save hundreds of lives, cheaply and easily, by donating money to the most cost-effective aid agencies. Most of us could save, relatively easily, 1350 lives over our life-time. True, but, again, this is because we happen to find ourselves in special circumstances which are conducive to our providing great benefits, namely a huge global inequality, in which we are vastly better off than many of those who need our help. Also, we could accomplish these greatly beneficial deeds only because there are already in place, due to the work of many good-natured people, highly cost-affective [sic] aid agencies. Therefore, we cannot justifiably claim the *whole* credit for the lives saved by our donations.[4]

---

[4] Persson and Savulescu, "Getting Moral Enhancement Right", p. 125.

I am entirely unclear why claiming the "whole credit" might be a crucial point, but insofar as it is, the cases are isomorphic. First, chances or opportunities have to exist to be taken, and we are seldom entirely responsible for creating the opportunities we take as well as for taking them. Opportunities are often, as the name implies, "opportunistic". So although the opportunity for doing good by giving aid, requires other things to be handily in place, so do opportunities for evil. To take P&S's own example, my ability to kill by driving my car into innocent bystanders is contingent upon *my happening to find myself in special circumstances which are conducive to my doing great harm*, namely my living within driving distance of a suitable crowd of such bystanders. Also it is only possible because *there are already in place, due to the work of many good-natured people, highly cost-effective* motor cars for me to drive, gas stations for me to fill the cars in, roads kindly built to facilitate my murderous instincts, etc., etc. And of course I can only do all this because I have the good fortune to *live in densely populated areas*, abounding with good natured and patient crowds just waiting for me to plough into them! I, for one, certainly can't take the whole credit for all of this, kind as it is of P&S to implausibly endow me and others of their readers with this degree of power.

Before I seize further murderous opportunities and take my car out for a spin towards Oxford let us return to the issue of moral or rather theoretical symmetry between causing death and saving lives.

9.2 How Much is Enough Moral Enhancement?

I have to say I see no relevant differences between the two cases P&S present and I am also sure that we are all modest enough only to claim the appropriate degree of credit for what we do or for what the characters in our examples are capable of. However, P&S have another big problem in maintaining, as they do, that there is a necessary or structural and, more importantly, substantial asymmetry between our capacity to do harm and in particular to kill, on the one hand, and our capacity to do good and in particular to save lives, on the other. This problem arises because P&S have nailed their colours to the mast of moral bioenhancement precisely because of this alleged asymmetry and because they see moral enhancement as required in order to prevent or indeed forestall the sort of apocalyptic harms that the village monster or the village idiot might, through monstrosity or idiocy, perpetrate upon a gullible public. If moral enhancement might be capable of this trick, or even if P&S think it might, then they must also think that both in principle and in fact that it is easy enough to save a large number of lives by this means.

Most significantly, if it wasn't in principle as easy to do good as to do harm, then the P&S argument for moral enhancement would be proportionally reduced in power and attractiveness. P&S seem not to have noticed that since moral bioenhancement is recommended by them precisely because of its allegedly crucial role in forestalling disaster, its success in this role will be proportionate to the extent to which they are wrong about the relative ease of preventing harm rather than doing good, about the relative ease of ending lives rather than saving them.

I use the term "easy" because although it may be very difficult (possibly impossible) to develop a reliable drug-based moral enhancer, once developed (like the motor car in the P&S example) it will be "easy peasy" to do instantly an immense power of good. That is why P&S have espoused moral enhancement so enthusiastically and it is also why they cannot have their cake and eat it too.

But there is another problem here. P&S believe that the world is particularly threatened because just one maniac or idiot might, given the immensely powerful and easily acquired destructive technologies that are increasingly readily accessible, destroy the world forever. For this reason, drastic preventive measures, namely universal moral enhancement are required.[5] But the task of developing, let alone universally distributing, these preventive measures is, to say the least, somewhat ambitious. Remember their radical solution is prompted by the possibility of just one outlier, one village idiot, destroying everything.

As P&S have insisted:

Even if only a tiny fraction of humanity is immoral enough to want to cause large scale harm by weapons of mass destruction in their possession, there are bound to be some such people in a huge human population, as on Earth, unless humanity is extensively morally enhanced . . .[6]

---

[5] Ingmar Persson and Julian Savulescu, "The Perils of Cognitive Enhancement and the Urgent Imperative to Enhance the Moral Character of Humanity", *Journal of Applied Philosophy*, vol. 25, no. 3 (2008): 162–77.

[6] Persson and Savulescu, "The Perils of Cognitive Enhancement", p. 174.

The remedy therefore must be more than extensive to do the trick; it must be universal and exceptionless. Even if the eventual moral enhancement could be applied as easily as via, for example, the oral administration of something on a sugar lump, we know from experience with the polio vaccine that it would be impossible to ensure anything like universal coverage. Moreover, unlike with vaccination, there will not be the benefits of 'herd immunity' to help mask deficits in coverage. The trick has been, by sufficiently extensive vaccination, to wipe out the disease itself.

I must continue to make clear that I have no objection to moral enhancement, or what P&S now call moral bioenhancement if, firstly it works, and secondly, if methods of moral bioenhancement do not counter-productively block alternative modalities of mitigating harm and doing good. My fear is that most of the evidence so far adduced for moral bioenhancement seems to indicate that it will fail to enhance morality and do good "all things considered".[7] I could be wrong about this of course, but that is why we must not use one strategy if there is a danger of it blocking another more promising one.

P&S seem to agree with this because they now say, as if I had ever denied such an approach:

But why should we bet on one against the other? Why can't we have both? Why can't we have scientific research accelerated by cognitive enhancement, but channel some of it towards finding means of moral bioenhancement?[8]

Oh why, oh why indeed can't we? I, of course, think we can, but I have to admit having been grossly and perversely misled by P&S themselves. In their original paper[9] P&S specifically conclude:

Even if only a tiny fraction of humanity is immoral enough to want to cause large scale harm by weapons of mass destruction in their possession, there are bound

---

[7] John Harris, "What It's Like to be Good", *Cambridge Quarterly of Healthcare Ethics*, vol. 21, no. 3 (2012): 293–305. See also John Harris and Sarah Chan, "Moral Behaviour is Not What It Seems", *Proceedings of the National Academy of Sciences USA*, Early Edition (2010): <http://www.pnas.org/cgi/doi/10.1073/pnas.1015001107>; Sarah Chan and John Harris, "Moral Enhancement and Prosocial Behaviour", *Journal of Medical Ethics*, vol. 37, no. 3 (2011): 130–1; John Harris, "'Ethics is for Bad Guys!': Putting the 'Moral' into Moral Enhancement", *Bioethics*, vol. 27, no. 3 (2013): 169–73.

[8] Persson and Savulescu, "Getting Moral Enhancement Right", p. 128.

[9] Persson and Savulescu, "The Perils of Cognitive Enhancement", p. 174.

to be some such people in a huge human population, as on Earth, unless humanity is extensively morally enhanced . . .

A moral enhancement of the magnitude required to ensure that this will not happen is not sufficiently possible at present and is not likely to be possible in the near future.

Therefore, the progress of science is in one respect for the worse by making likelier the misuse of ever more effective weapons of mass destruction, and this badness is increased if scientific progress is speeded up by cognitive enhancement, until effective means of moral enhancement are found and applied.

Admittedly they say "in one respect" the progress of science is for the worse, but they discuss no other senses in which the progress of science is in any way for the better given the dangers that preoccupy them. I have argued elsewhere that science is our chief hope for the future of humankind, and in particular for the discovery of methods of blocking doomsday scenarios of the sort imagined by P&S.[10] Given the significance of the apocalyptic threats, and the whole direction of their paper being the need urgently to combat these threats, I took them to be recommending that we put on hold both or even attempt to reverse the progress of science and cognitive enhancement pending the development of moral enhancement. Indeed, Elizabeth Fenton was equally comprehensively deceived by the above claim, pointing out "it is difficult not to take [Persson's and Savulescu's pessimism] to imply that unless and until we further understand moral enhancement, we should try to slow scientific progress".[11] I am glad to be reassured that P&S, like me, are in favour of pursuing research into all forms of enhancement even though, in their view, these different methods may be mutually antagonistic.

9.3 Unenhanced Dichotomies

P&S quote me correctly as saying: "The space between knowing the good and doing the good is a region entirely inhabited by freedom." And then present this dichotomy:

Suppose, first, that our freedom is compatible with it being fully determined whether or not we shall do what we take to be good. Then a judicious use of

---

[10] John Harris, *Enhancing Evolution* (Princeton and Oxford: Princeton University Press, 2007).

[11] Elizabeth Fenton, "The Perils of Failing to Enhance: A Response to Persson and Savulescu", *Journal of Medical Ethics*, vol. 36, no. 3 (2010): 148–51, at p. 149.

moral bioenhancement techniques will not reduce our freedom; it will simply make it the case that we are more often, perhaps always, determined to do what we take to be good. We would then act as a morally perfect person now would act. Suppose, on the other hand, that we are free only because, by nature, we are not fully determined to do what we take to be good. Then moral bioenhancement cannot be fully effective because its effectiveness is limited by our freedom in this indeterministic sense. So, irrespective of whether determinism or indeterminism in the realm of human action is true, moral bioenhancement will not curtail our freedom.

P&S seem to be suggesting that this dichotomy somehow demonstrates that the alternatives divide without remainder in a way that demonstrates that I must be wrong.[12] This horse won't run! They are assuming in the first paragraph that all methods by which actions might be "fully determined" are the same from the perspective of the room left for the role of choice. I have expressed doubts about the extent to which some chemical and biological ways of altering the emotions and other springs of actions leave room for choice in the way that many believe the thesis that all events including mental events are caused leaves room among those causes for choices. So it does not follow from the fact that either some form of determinism is true or none is, (the dichotomy) and that determinism *can be* compatible with free will, that absolutely any form of determinism *must be* so compatible; and hence if moral bioenhancement involves determinism it is necessarily not antagonistic to freedom. P&S and I are discussing precisely whether or not there will be some forms of moral bioenhancement that will leave room for freedom. I am sure there can be such; I have argued, however, that many of the forms currently being canvassed as promising do not in fact augur well for the survival of either liberty or indeed for the survival of rational strategies for seeing that good triumphs "all things considered".

I think that the P&S choice of a combination of altruism and a sense of justice is as good a choice as any for core moral dispositions although one must be clear that if so, "a sense of justice" is an extremely theory-laden idea in a way that simple "do-gooding" may not be. My concern is first to avoid the elimination of deliberation from our understanding of what makes for a moral judgement, to avoid methods which bypass reflection

---

[12] Such "unenhanced dichotomies", in less politically correct times, were called "false dichotomies".

and deliberation. Some philosophers, like Tom Douglas, have regarded the avoidance of deliberation as an advantage:

The distinctive feature of emotional moral enhancement is that, once the enhancement has been initiated, there is no further need for cognition: emotions are modified directly.[13]

Douglas glossed this idea in a later paper in which he appears to have kept to this view.[14]

It is unclear whether or not P&S also regard this as an advantage of moral bioenhancement, but whether or not they do, it is likely that the currently foreseen methods of moral bioenhancement will in fact operate in this way.[15]

Secondly, current chemical and biological methods of intervention which have been taken to have implications for moral enhancement are targeted on so-called "pro-social" emotions which tend to operate on what can be immediately seen, heard, and felt, rather than on what we know might be happening beyond what we can immediately see, hear, and feel. Such methods may distort the moral priorities which we would have if we considered more and felt less. I do not think P&S and I are, all things considered, so far apart; and contrary to what they obviously believe, I have no antipathy at all to moral enhancement per se.

9.4 Moral Reasoning and Moral Judgement

Carl Sagan has reported that he is:

often asked the question, "Do you think there is extra-terrestrial intelligence?" I give the standard arguments—there are a lot of places out there, and use the word billions, and so on. And then I say it would be astonishing to me if there

---

[13] Tom Douglas, Unpublished manuscript draft for "Moral Enhancement via Direct Emotion Modulation: A Reply to John Harris", *Bioethics*, vol. 27, no. 3 (2013): 160–8.

[14] Tom Douglas, "Enhancing Moral Conformity and Enhancing Moral Worth", *Neuroethics*, vol. 7, no. 1 (2014): 75–91. See p. 76.

[15] Molly J. Crockett, Luke Clark, Marc D. Hauser, and Trevor W. Robbins, "Serotonin Selectively Influences Moral Judgment and Behavior through Effects on Harm Aversion", *Proceedings of the National Academy of Sciences USA*, vol. 107, no. 40 (2010): 17433–8; Molly J. Crockett, Luke Clark, Marc D. Hauser, and Trevor W. Robbins, "Reply to Harris and Chan: Moral Judgment is More than Rational Deliberation", *Proceedings of the National Academy of Sciences of the United States of America*, vol. 107, no. 50 (2010): E184; Harris and Chan, "Moral Behaviour is Not What It Seems". Daniel M. Bartels and David A. Pizarro, "The Mismeasure of Morals: Antisocial Personality Traits Predict Utilitarian Responses to Moral Dilemmas", *Cognition*, vol. 121, no. 1 (2011): 154–61. In this paper moral judgements are treated as if they were not deliberative in any important sense.

weren't extra-terrestrial intelligence, but of course there is as yet no compelling evidence for it. And then I'm asked, "Yeah, but what do you really think?" I say, "I just told you what I really think." "Yeah, but what's your gut feeling?" But I try not to think with my gut.[16]

Well, in a modest way I try not to do ethics with my gut either, and if at all possible I would like my successors not to be determined by some well-meaning philosophers to have to do ethics that way, or to think that they needed no longer to ask themselves if what they were conditioned, or determined, to think right is indeed right?

To believe that emotions can deliver answers to moral dilemmas or generate moral judgements is like believing that the gut is an organ of thought, or one that can answer complex, combined theoretical and empirical, questions. Ethical judgements involve, almost always, a combination of evidence and argument and where this combination becomes disjoint, they, at the very least, involve judgement. By judgement is meant something involving reasoning and argument towards a conclusion, towards a "judgement" properly so called. Ethical judgements cannot, literally cannot, be felt. There is no sense organ for such a feeling. They can of course be stipulated rather than judged of, but stipulation butters no parsnips, and only well buttered parsnips cut the mustard in ethics.

The reason for this is easily illustrated. Moral dilemmas present a choice, a parting of the ways at a junction. The resolution of a moral dilemma requires a moral reason to travel one road and not the other, not just any old reason, not simply an arbitrary election or random choice between one pathway and another, nor even a poetic or practical reason. There may be many reasons to travel one road rather than another, but only some of them are moral reasons. And only the exercise of moral reason can lead to a moral judgement. The roads may both involve morally consequential journeys, journeys that make a moral difference, to the traveller or to the world. But even morally consequential journeys can be embarked upon for frivolous or trivial or prejudiced or prejudicial reasons or for no reason at all. Moral judgement, and hence moral enhancement leads to better moral decision-making, but not necessarily to better moral outcomes.

---

[16] Carl Sagan, "The Burden of Skepticism", *Skeptical Inquirer*, vol. 12 (Fall 1987): <http://www.positiveatheism.org/writ/saganbur.htm>, accessed 12 October 2011.

Robert Frost eloquently identified one dilemma of choice where there seems little or nothing to choose between different paths and yet one knows that the choice will prove hugely consequential in the long term. Here is the last verse:

> I shall be telling this with a sigh
> Somewhere ages and ages hence:
> Two roads diverged in a wood, and I
> I took the one less traveled by,
> And that has made all the difference.[17]

In fact we know that Robert Frost sent this poem to his friend the poet Wilfred Owen and it seems to have played an important role in resolving a life-changing dilemma, convincing Owen to join the army, a decision that resulted in his death only a week from the end of the First World War on 4 November 1918.

There are many reasons why this (and in principle any) choice between two roads, taken, as the text makes clear, for no decisive reason, moral or otherwise, might prove hugely consequential and indeed "make all the difference" including all the moral difference, even "ages and ages hence". But a decision that makes a moral difference is not for that reason a moral decision, nor is a dilemma the resolution of which has moral consequences for that reason a moral dilemma.[18] As Ronald Dworkin[19] has convincingly shown, moral judgements command a special respect which is due to them partly because they are taken to reflect the considered values of the individual making them, and partly because moral judgements have to meet certain minimum standards of evidence and argument which exclude a number of disqualifying features. Such disqualifying features include gut reactions, and instinctive or automatic responses. Moreover moral judgements are required to be distinguishable from prejudices, arbitrary preferences, personal tastes, arguments or conclusions based on manifest self-interest or partiality, or arising from a personal emotional response, e.g. "they make me sick!", "it

---

[17] Robert Frost, "Road Not Taken": <http://www.poets.org/viewmedia.php/prmMID/15717>, accessed 10 October 2011.

[18] John Harris, Introduction: "The Scope and Importance of Bioethics", in John Harris (ed.), *Bioethics*. Oxford Readings in Philosophy Series (Oxford: Oxford University Press, 2001).

[19] Ronald Dworkin, *Taking Rights Seriously* (London: Duckworth, 1977), Chapter 9.

is disgusting!" and the like. Finally someone claiming to act out of moral principle or on the basis of moral judgement must be able to explain just what is wrong with the conduct to which he objects or right about the decision she endorses.

As I have argued earlier (in Chapters 1, 2, and 3),[20] exactly as not just any judgement about things in which science is interested is "scientific" so not just any judgements about things with which morality is concerned are moral judgements. There may of course be argument about just what more is required in each case. I have, following Dworkin, suggested some minimal standards for morality; these severally, and perhaps even jointly, are certainly contestable. But that some such standards are required is not I suggest open to doubt. Something must distinguish morality from other normative systems or systems of belief more generally. And just as not all rules about things that interest the law are legal rules so not all judgements about things that interest morality are moral judgements and not all normative systems are either legal or moral (dress codes in the workplace or the 'laws' of cricket). To be sure, the elements of any particular legal system, or code of conduct, may be contested jurisprudence; but uncertainty does not mean "anything goes", uncertainty almost always has parameters which are well understood just as some uncertainty about linguistic meaning, "ambiguity", is not total uncertainty, but uncertainty within a range.[21]

Tom Douglas invites us to think about Bryony:

Bryony is a student from a wealthy family. She suspects she ought to do more to help the global poor. She does occasionally do something to help, for example, giving small amounts to support famine relief when approached by charities, but most of the time, the world's most unfortunate are far from her thoughts, and when they do cross her mind, she has trouble drumming up the sort of sympathy that might motivate greater sacrifices on her part. In an attempt to remedy this, she sets up her television so that it regularly displays disturbing and graphic images of the effects of poverty, though for such brief periods that she does not consciously recognise them. Nevertheless, through subliminal effects, the images do increase her feelings of sympathy, and these feelings stimulate her to make a large donation to Oxfam.[22]

---

[20] See also Harris, "What It's Like to be Good".

[21] William Empson, *Seven Types of Ambiguity*, 3rd edition (London: Chatto & Windus, 1970, first published 1930). The range in question may be indefinite but it is not infinite.

[22] Douglas, "Enhancing Moral Conformity and Enhancing Moral Worth", p. 78.

It seems to me that Douglas and indeed Savulescu and Persson who use this or similar examples are taking an excessively (one might say "obsessively") individualist view of the way to solve, not Bryony's problem—that is indeed a problem—but rather the way to solve or help solve global poverty. I have argued that ethics is for bad guys (Chapter 7); the good don't need ethics and neither does Bryony. What she needs is determination, not goodness. But more important than the needs of bad guys, who perhaps we should disregard as beyond the pale of our moral concern, is addressing the problem of global poverty which it is, I suggest, insane to leave to personal altruism.

We should not worry too much about Bryony's weakness of will! What we need in order to solve, or even help mitigate, global poverty is a global solution and this must be attempted at a minimum at state level, and probably at an international or global level. It is clear we cannot provide health care "free at the point of need"[23] by private altruism. What we need is, at minimum, a national health care system (like the NHS in the UK) delivered centrally using taxation (to which all contribute) to fund it. We need this, and other care and social welfare measures, precisely because we know that altruism so often fails (perhaps because of a combination of human weakness in the form not least of weakness of will, but also because of the human weakness of not being able to drum up much sympathy for the ugly and unsavoury or for those out of sight and out of mind). We cannot deliver health care "free at the point of need" except at a national level, nor can we provide social security, and other social services including for example fire, police, ambulance, and defence forces in such a way either.

In a real sense it is gross self-indulgence, not to mention self-defeating, to try to address these big problems at the level of individual morality. Let's leave poor Chloe alone and think about addressing these important problems at the level of policy and indeed of government or better, at a combined governmental, truly international, level. This is what P&S would have to do to implement moral bioenhancement, and if we all did more to ensure that governments acted effectively on global poverty, climate change, education, population control, disease prevention, clean water and the like we might not even need to consider threats to liberty of

---

[23] A phrase used by successive UK governments to describe the aspirations for care to be delivered by the NHS.

the sort I believe that some forms of moral enhancement would inevitably entail. We don't need moral enhancement to see the force of this. What do we need?

9.5 Power to the People

Neglected, as far as serious consideration in the literature is concerned, are the possibly beneficial effects of increasing affluence at least on the disposition to resort to political use of weapons of mass destruction. Attention was first drawn to one such effect by Bertrand Russell in 1930, but so far it has not received the attention it deserves.

Russell, in an insightful essay entitled "Is Happiness Still Possible"[24] was bemoaning the apathy of the West in the interwar years when contrasted with what he saw as the dynamism of the "young intelligentsia" in India, China, and Japan:

Cynicism such as one finds very frequently among the most highly educated young men and women of the West results from the combination of comfort with powerlessness. Powerlessness makes people feel that nothing is worth doing, and comfort makes the painfulness of that feeling just endurable.

There is an important sense in which we want to encourage the sort of cynicism which makes people too apathetic to resort to violent political action and it may be that the promotion of comfort and satisfaction with life is a more reliable and even more morally respectable way of achieving this than the sorts of moral enhancement that might deprive us of free will. If we couple universal education with the eradication of poverty and more, increasing affluence, we will I believe be doing the most promising thing as far as moral enhancement goes. That does not mean that we should forgo other means, but it is self-defeating to use methods that undermine the very capacities required both for moral reflection and judgement but also for moral progress.

---

[24] Bertrand Russell, *The Conquest of Happiness* (London: Unwin Books, 1964, first published 1930).

10

Mind Reading and Mind Misreading

10.1 Introduction

The idea, the possibility of reading the mind, from the outside, or indeed even from the inside, has exercised humanity from the earliest times. Perhaps the earliest reference to mind reading in Western literature occurs in Homer. Hector's last words as he lies dying at the hand of Achilles takes up our theme:

Hector of the flashing helmet spoke to him once more at the point of death. "How well I know you and can read your mind" he said.[1]

If, and to the extent that we could, read other minds this would be a powerful tool in moral enhancement not least because it might enable the criminal law to anticipate crimes in advance of their commission and resolve vexed problems of intent. Recent advances in neuroscience have offered some, probably remote, prospect of improved access, but a different branch of technology seems to offer the most promising and the most daunting prospect for both mind reading and mind misreading. We should bear in mind that you can't have the possibility of reading without the possibility of misreading.

A working party of the Royal Society in 2010–11, on which I served, examined these issues, and although that working party emphatically concluded[2] that the case was not proven for the use of brain state

---

[1] Homer, *The Iliad* (Harmondsworth: Penguin Books, 1966), Book XXII, pp. 403–73, at p. 406.

[2] The Royal Society, *Brain Waves Module 4: Neuroscience and the Law*. ISBN: 978-0-85403-932-6, December 2011: <http://royalsociety.org/policy/projects/brain-waves/responsibility-law/>, accessed 7 June 2014. I was a member of this working party so declare an interest and some small responsibility for its findings.

evidence particularly as to intent, in criminal trials, we also noted that this situation may well change in the future and should be kept under review.[3]

Soul-searching is not identical with mind reading, nor is mind reading identical with (even if it were possible to achieve such a thing), a complete description of brain activity. An analogue here may be the relationship between genetics and epigenetics. Many neuroscientists and philosophers of neuroscience seem stuck in an era equivalent to genetic essentialism and oblivious to the era of epigenetics and its cerebral equivalent. Maybe desires, motives, intentions, and attitudes, and both external and first-person access to these, stand to a map of the brain or a description of brain activity, as understanding the behaviour or functioning of a creature stands to the map of its genome. We know from contemporary epigenetics that the behaviour of genes, gene expression, is influenced by the coding of the genes but also by environmental factors as well as, for example, being modulated by patterns of inhibitors and promoters other than DNA, that are set up within the cell and are self-perpetuating.

As we noted in Chapter 6, Wittgenstein famously remarked in connection with establishing the reference, the object referred to in speech: "If God had looked into our minds he would not have been able to see there of whom we were speaking."[4] Why wouldn't he? If we consider the questions: is this murder? or is this rape? the answers to questions such as these are not to be found in states of the brain, not least because in the case of rape, the consent or otherwise of the other party is not to be found in the brain state of the putative rapist and in the case of murder, whether or not the act of killing might constitute self-defence is likewise not to be found in brain states.

---

[3] See also Jana Bufkin and Vickie Luttrell, "Neuroimaging and Studies of Aggressive and Violent Behavior", *Trauma Violence Abuse*, vol. 6, no. 2 (2005): 176–91; Adrian Raine and Yaling Yang, "Neural Foundations to Moral Reasoning and Antisocial Behavior", *Social Cognitive and Affective Neuroscience*, vol. 1, no. 3 (2006): 203–13; Nigel Eastman and Colin Campbell, "Neuroscience and Legal Determination of Criminal Responsibility", *Nature Reviews Neuroscience*, vol. 7, no. 4 (2006): 311–18; Teneille R. Brown and Emily R. Murphy, "Through a Scanner Darkly: Functional Neuroimaging as Evidence of a Criminal Defendant's Past Mental States", *Stanford Law Review*, vol. 62, no. 4 (2010): 1119–208.

[4] Ludwig Wittgenstein, *Philosophical Investigations*, trans. G. E. M. Anscombe (Oxford: Basil Blackwell, 1968), Part IIxi at p. 217. Since this is a translation I have taken the liberty of improving upon Elizabeth Anscombe's grasp of English grammar.

Relatedly, we have the illusion that memories are traces of experienced events, thoughts, and feelings brought to mind sometime after the experiences themselves. But while memory is pretty certainly due to brain states, two further 'things' are not. First whether what we remember actually happened and therefore whether or not it is in fact a 'memory' is one hypothesis. The second hypothesis is that our memory is a recalled trace of earlier experiences including thoughts and feelings occasioned by something in the world. We simply do not reliably know whether apparent memories are simply 'memories' of a previous memory, which itself involved many hypotheses about events both in the mind and elsewhere in the world.

10.2 Mind Reading

Mind reading and the relationship between the face, particularly the eyes, and the contents of the mind or indeed of the soul has been and remains a fascination for humankind. This preoccupation reflects a fact about human beings. We want to read minds, including our own, we want this so that we understand what kind of person the bearer[5] of the mind is, who we have to deal with, how they are likely to behave, what they want, what they are likely to do and what they have done. And we need to know these things about ourselves quite as much as about others. What manner of man am I? What sort of woman are you? Mind reading of course would also reveal moral qualities as well as intentions. In addition to being a powerful moral enhancer, mind reading, if and insofar as it can be done, would be a powerful cognitive enhancer and, like all knowledge, a significant source of power.

The image of the eyes or the face as windows into mind or the soul often plays a seminal role in the imagery we use to discuss the project of mind reading. Perhaps the earliest references to the eyes as windows on the soul come from Cicero, who is here expanding on the nature of oratory—formal speech-making:

---

[5] This turn of phrase is borrowed from Shakespeare's Brutus: "Think not, thou noble Roman, That ever Brutus will go bound to Rome. He bears too great a mind." *Julius Caesar*, Act 5, Scene 1. All Shakespeare quotations are from The Arden Shakespeare, *Complete Works*, ed. Richard Proudfoot, Ann Thomson, and David Scott Kastan (Walton-on-Thames: Thomas Nelson and Sons, 1998).

the countenance itself is entirely dominated by the eyes; . . . For delivery [oratory] is wholly the concern of the feelings, and these are mirrored by the face and expressed by the eyes.[6]

But in *Macbeth* we find Duncan decisively rejecting any idea of either the eyes or the face revealing much of forensic use:

There's no art
To find the mind's construction in the face[7]

This emphatic rejection of what we might think of as intuitive mind reading is probably right, and as noted, for the present also goes for neuroscientific attempts to open a different window on the soul. But there exists a powerful technology that is persuading many that mind reading and perhaps so far more usually mind misreading is already with us. This is the access provided by "the cloud" to any digitized material.

I will use the term "the cloud" to stand generically for the Internet but also for indeed anything recorded on digitizing kit that can be recovered and made explicit despite apparent deletion. This goes beyond the standard equivalence of the cloud and the Internet, but is I think justified as we shall see. It is, I will claim, the cloud that has replaced the eyes, or the face or indeed the brain as the most potent avenue of access to the human mind and perhaps also to synthetic minds.

10.3   Thinking and Feeling in the Cloud

Life in the cloud is immortal and omnipresent and, almost, as replete with feelings as our own dear lives.[8] We must now accept that our words, and to an extent, our actions and thoughts are permanently "in the cloud" and accessible to anyone and everyone. Of course thoughts and actions are as open to interpretation as words and always as ambiguous. As William Empson famously remarked, "in a sufficiently extended sense any prose statement could be called ambiguous".[9]

---

[6] Cicero, *De Oratore* III, 221. *Cicero On The Orator*, trans. H. Rackham. Loeb Classical Library (Cambridge, MA and London: Harvard University Press, 1942), p. 177.

[7] William Shakespeare, *Macbeth*, Act 1, Scene 4, lines 12ff, p. 775.

[8] Here again discussion follows lines elaborated in John Harris, "Life in the Cloud and Freedom of Speech", *Journal of Medical Ethics*, vol. 39, no. 5 (2012): 307–11.

[9] William Empson, *Seven Types of Ambiguity* (London: Chatto & Windus, 1970, first published 1930), Chapter 1.

As I suggested elsewhere concerning the existence of the cloud:

This is a game-changing [innovation], and indeed constitutes a very dangerous turn of events. Not only is it a possible restriction, not just on free speech but on the possibility of sober, or even informed or nuanced discussion, it also constitutes perhaps the final erosion of the distinction between speaking and acting, and indeed between thought and action, and may have already expanded the scope of the "reckless" part of the coupling of "reckless" with "endangerment" to the point of no return.

This is because, not only do we have no knowledge or control over who will have access to our words and in what circumstances, we do not even have any control over how they will be edited, sensationalised, decontextualised, bowdlerised or otherwise distorted. We must be always aware of the potentially limitless scope, and indeed duration, of what we say.[10]

An example of the radical expansion of access to our words is provided by a comment made on a news story recently, which spread in an amazing way.

"Companies like Novartis should not be in the position to block moves to more cost-effective treatments in order to maximize their profits," said John Harris of the Institute for Science Ethics and Innovation at the University of Manchester.

This comment was made in a press release; Reuters put it on the wires and the report subsequently received "Page Views: 31,088,501, Unique Visitors: 4,572,149."[11] More than 4.5 million different individuals accessed this comment online and in addition to the "hits" on the Web and visitors to the site this remark was reported in 278 separate national and local news outlets, both broadcast and print.

As the Chairman of Google, Eric Schmidt, has remarked:

The fact that there is no delete button on the internet forces public policy choices we had never imagined.[12]

---

[10] Harris, "Life in the Cloud and Freedom of Speech", p. 308.

[11] 01/05/2012 Outlet Name: Reuters—Source: <http://www.vocuspr.com/uk> (The University of Manchester's media monitoring service—subscription required for access); ZURICH/LONDON (Reuters)—Swiss drug-maker Novartis is challenging the use of a cheap alternative to its eye drug Lucentis in parts of Britain, sparking a row over cost versus safety in treating a common cause of blindness.

[12] <http://www.guardian.co.uk/technology/2012/may/23/google-fund-teachers-computer-science-uk>, accessed 3 June 2014.

Recently a landmark European Court ruling[13] on the right to be forgotten may indeed lead to the removal of items of personal data from particular sites or local search engines but will not mean that the relevant data have been entirely expunged from the cloud, nor from databases nor computers nor rendered inaccessible.

Nuance is not something the Internet does well, and neither is "the cloud" well adapted to audience selection. John Stuart Mill famously finessed freedom of speech,[14] and indeed of assembly, in the following terms:

No one pretends that actions should be as free as opinions. On the contrary, even opinions lose their immunity when the circumstances in which they are expressed are such as to constitute their expression a positive instigation to some mischievous act. An opinion that corn-dealers are starvers of the poor, or that private property is robbery, ought to be unmolested when simply circulated through the press, but may justly incur punishment when delivered orally to an excited mob assembled before the house of a corn-dealer, or when handed about among the same mob in the form of a placard. Acts, of whatever kind, which without justifiable cause, do harm to others, may be, and in the more important cases absolutely require to be, controlled by the unfavourable sentiments, and, when needful, by the active interference of mankind.[15]

We now, it seems, have to talk or write as if we might always be addressing a violent mob assembled before the equivalent of "the house of a corn-dealer". For with smart phones and other portable devices in the hands of who knows who, who knows where or in what circumstances, that is just what we might be doing when writing, even in the sober pages of a book published by Oxford University Press.

In the cloud, words and indeed images and sounds exist, as far as we know, forever, in all places and all times. This is the immortality that some have dreamed of.[16] It also further erodes the traditional distinction

---

[13] European Court of Justice Judgment, Case C-131/12 ECLI:EU:C:2014:616 13 May 2014. Full text available at: <http://curia.europa.eu/juris/document/document.jsf.jsessionid= 9ea7d2dc30d5cfb78416675447019937a19787b77870.e34KaxiLc3qMb40Rch0SaxuNbxr0?text=& docid=152065&pageIndex=0&doclang=EN&mode=req&dir=&occ=first&part=1&cid=124853>, accessed 6 June 2014; <http://www.bbc.co.uk/news/technology-27631001>, accessed 3 June 2014.

[14] Harris, "Life in the Cloud and Freedom of Speech".

[15] John Stuart Mill, *On Liberty* (1859), Chapter III, in Mary Warnock (ed.), *Utilitarianism* (London: Collins/Fontana, 1972), p. 184.

[16] John Harris, "Intimations of Immortality", *Science*, vol. 288, no. 5463 (2000): 59; John Harris, "Intimations of Immortality: The Ethics and Justice of Life Extending Therapies", in

between words and action and possibly also between thoughts and words, since speculations may be taken to be proposals and exposure of the weakness of an argument *against* something may be taken to be an argument *for* it. This gives scope for radical misunderstanding and misrepresentation. But perhaps even more important than the fact that our words, actions, and thoughts are forever in the cloud is the fact that, insofar as they are digitized they can in principle be accessed by anyone with the requisite skills. As Bruce Schneier made clear in an oral presentation to the Royal Society,[17] anything submitted or recorded online would be permanently in the cloud, accessible to anyone (like himself) knowledgeable enough to access them. Moreover, as Schneier noted, "all the research is being done on computers" and "any computer can be hacked, not most, any!"[18] This is why I include all digitized material in my rather nebulous definition of the cloud.

In the cloud we have a permanent, accessible, and in principle freely available archive of everything we have ever recorded digitally.

What has so far been generally overlooked is that this constitutes the most comprehensive gateway to the soul (or way of constructing an alternative soul ab initio) ever discovered, in principle available to all and permanently accessible.

In short, we already have massive capacity for "mind reading" and hence of mind misreading from which there is no effective defence, and to which most of us are exposed. Here, we speak of those aspects of our minds and your mind that have been digitized, that is, put into computer memory or onto the Internet—into the cloud. There is no defence, anything that has ever been on a computer let alone been e-mailed or stored in the cloud can be read and downloaded and that access cannot be prevented.

If we think about what "data" most of us have consigned to the cloud the list can be alarming. Most of us now write on digitizing kit: computers, tablets, phones; most of us also write and receive e-mails, tweets, and so on, many have a "web presence"—a Facebook or Twitter account, or a website—and many also keep their diaries and appointments in

Michael Freeman (ed.), *Current Legal Problems* (Oxford: Oxford University Press, 2002), pp. 65–97.

[17] <http://www.voiceprompt.co.uk/royalsociety/030412/#>, accessed 25 June 2014.
[18] <https://royalsociety.org/events/2012/viruses/>, accessed 3 June 2014.

electronic media. Moreover the cloud contains a record of websites we have "visited"—of things we have ordered online, many of us fill in our tax returns online, pay fines online, visit online medical services like NHS Direct, we look up medical conditions online, order drugs and services many of which may be unavailable or even illegal in our own countries . . . the list is as large as our imagination and as inventive as Google's algorithms.

We should be clear, much of this will contain the substance of what we believe on many matters, what we are minded to do or to consider doing, what we have done, including elements of our desires and fantasies, interests, what we know and don't know, our preoccupations, activities, patterns of behaviour, of purchasing, of expenditure, what are the objects of our gaze and more or less reliable inferences can be drawn about what sort of gaze it is.

Some aspects of this are starting to arouse interest.[19] People using the Internet are becoming increasingly aware of the dangers of images and things they say on Facebook or other websites; perhaps aided, ironically, by the proliferation of news feeds and novel forms of communication provided by the cloud. The rise of highly visible 'cyberstalking' applications such as *Creepy*,[20] which aggregates geolocation data attached to various tweets, updates, photos, and the like from any chosen poster and generates a map of the subject's whereabouts; and extensive media coverage focused on cyber-bullying,[21] with hundreds of tragic and often upsetting stories doing the rounds have attracted attention. Charities, victims, and the families of victims of these dangers have started campaigns to publicize them[22] and to offer advice and assistance.

---

[19] In the following sections I am again massively indebted to David Lawrence for insights and for crucial research.

[20] Although developed in 2011 ostensibly as a means of raising awareness of the ease of cyber stalking, Creepy is still available freely from <http://creepy.en.softonic.com/>, accessed 6 June 2014.

[21] A simple Internet search for "examples of cyberbullying on social networking sites" raises around 368,000 results from media outlet sites. They are perhaps best summed up in this article from the BBC: <http://www.bbc.co.uk/news/education-23727673>, accessed 6 June 2014.

[22] Such as: <http://deletecyberbullying.eu/>, <http://www.nasuwt.org.uk/Whatsnew/Campaigns/StopCyberbullying/NASUWT_002654>, and <http://www.athinline.org/All>, accessed 6 June 2014.

Research suggests that among users in what is generally regarded as the most vulnerable group, pre-teens and early teenagers, there is a "[belief] in the value of online privacy", and that:

educational opportunities regarding internet privacy and computer security as well as concerns from other reference groups (e.g., peer, teacher, and parents) play an important role in positively affecting the Internet users' protective behavior regarding online privacy.[23]

The rising awareness of the public and the willingness to respond to the potential dangers of the cloud are perhaps well illustrated by a recent petition against a newly announced Facebook feature, which would "let it listen to our conversations and surroundings through our own phones' microphone."[24]

10.4 One Recent Example

A recent news story is particularly telling. On 21 March 2014 the BBC reported that: "[a] woman who threw acid in the face of a friend while wearing a veil as a disguise has been jailed for 12 years." The conviction of Mary Konye for this assault on Naomi Oni was widely reported.[25] The victim had been disbelieved by police, they had examined her laptop hard drive and found that she had "looked at plastic surgery websites" and at news features concerning Katie Piper. Katie Piper was a young woman who, in 2008, as *The Guardian* reported, "was raped by a man she'd met online. He then arranged for someone to throw acid in her face."[26] Armed with what they thought was evidence concerning Naomi Oni's state of mind, the police thought, or through lack of thought assumed, that this was evidence of her self-harming rather than, as proved to be true, or her being the victim of a malicious and vicious attack.[27]

---

[23] S. Chai, S. Bagchi-Sen, C. Morrell, H. Rao, and S. Upadhyaya, "Internet and Online Information Privacy: An Exploratory Study of Preteens and Early Teens", *IEEE Transactions on Professional Communication*, vol. 52, no. 2 (2009): 167–82.

[24] <http://action.sumofus.org/a/Facebook-app-taps-phones/?akid=5478.2614652.96-Mk1&rd=1&sub=fwd&t=2>, accessed 6 June 2014.

[25] <http://www.bbc.co.uk/news/uk-england-london-26680664>, accessed 9 June 2014.

[26] <http://www.theguardian.com/lifeandstyle/2012/jun/02/katie-piper-acid-attack-book>, accessed 9 June 2014.

[27] Naomi Oni Interviewed on BBC Radio 4 Today, 24 March 2014: <http://www.bbc.co.uk/programmes/p01w49sq>, accessed 2 April 2014.

As the UK newspaper *The Daily Mirror* reported at the time of the assault on Ms Oni (25 February 2013): "Officers seized the 20-year-old's laptop after discovering she had viewed websites about acid burn victims before she was hurt."[28]

The police in this case were guilty of an error of inference, one of the most common errors to which humankind is subject. Moreover, the cloud simply contains data, often without context, almost always without other relevant information. For example the cloud is irony blind; it usually contains no data on the tone of voice. Often there is also no context. Remarks which may be nuanced in print, or for example in a public statement or speech, often appear in truncated form, without nuance on the Internet. I have watched while members of the audience at a public lecture he was giving have "tweeted" extracts onto the Internet which then appeared without the nuance or qualification that the lecture contained.[29]

It is true that those of us who publish, broadcast, speak publicly, etc. place our minds to an extent in the public domain where they may freely be 'read' by all and sundry. But most of us do so or do so potentially without realizing that that is what we have done or without realizing that set in a new context, without nuance, qualification, or other caveats the meaning will inevitably be not only distorted but sometimes corrupted beyond recognition.

More significant by far, all people who use devices that record or transmit digitally are, almost certainly, placing themselves, if not on public record, at least in a universally and permanently accessible public domain. This is a domain in which increasingly inferences will be drawn (conservatively or recklessly or anything in between), about what we think, feel, believe, wish for or intend, desire or dread. Some of the inferences drawn about us will be reasonable and accurate enough, and for the foreseeable future these will constitute the best available windows on the soul.

---

[28] <http://www.mirror.co.uk/news/uk-news/naomi-oni-acid-burns-victim-1729522#ixzz 347hivunu>.

[29] I originally wrote this chapter with my colleague and PhD student David Lawrence. A version of our co-authored paper appeared in *Cambridge Quarterly of Healthcare Ethics*, vol. 24, no. 2 (2015). David was principally responsible for the significant amount of research on the science of mind reading that that paper contained and for the sections of that paper which discussed this research. Although this chapter does not cover the same ground as David's research I have been considerably influenced and indeed inspired by David Lawrence throughout and also in revising our earlier paper for this chapter.

11

The Safety of the People

The office of the sovereign, be it a monarch or an assembly, consisteth in the end for which he was trusted with the sovereign power, namely the procuration of *the safety of the people*; to which he is obliged by the law of nature.

Thomas Hobbes, *Leviathan*[1]

A king's lot: to do good and be damned.

Marcus Aurelius, *Meditations*[2]

11.1 Introduction

In Chapter 2, I indicated that moral obligations can often be best discharged collectively. I suggested that:

The limitations of individual morality do not necessarily, however, apply collectively. The obligations we may owe to one another seem sometimes overwhelming, particularly when they are seen as involving negative responsibility (our responsibility for the consequences of omissions) as well as positive responsibility (our responsibility for the consequences of doings rather than simply of refrainings).[3] Mutual moral responsibilities may, however, be more realistic and achievable at a society or national level by such beings as are we, than they are at the individual level. Public services are a good example. Health, welfare, and national defence are unlikely to be effectively deliverable in modern societies by individual action or private initiatives. So that levels of altruism that are beyond the power of individuals may be effectively deliverable by governments or other social institutions. No individual can usually hope to "feed the poor", defend the weak, or "heal

[1] Thomas Hobbes, *Leviathan* (1651), ed. Michael Oakeshott (Oxford: Basil Blackwell, 1960), Part II, Chapter 30, p. 219.

[2] Marcus Aurelius, *Meditations*, trans. Martin Hammond, with an Introduction by Diskin Clay (London: Penguin Books, 2006), Book 7.36, p. 63.

[3] I wrote about acts and omissions extensively in my book *Violence and Responsibility* (London: Routledge & Kegan Paul, 1980).

the sick", but good social welfare and health services and infrastructure (whether publicly or privately funded) can and do, so far as this is possible at all.

Now is the moment to set out in more detail the basis of my optimism about both the varieties of goodness and the many ways in which we can rationally understand how to be good. In setting out now what I judge to be a well-established basis for collective or state responsibility for the safety of the people in all its forms, I will employ one classic version of what is often called "social contract theory". In doing so I should make clear that I see no tension between this and the theoretical basis which grounds and should guide us in practising enhancement including moral enhancement. That basis is an understanding of the generic nature of the good and the obligation to do as much good as we can, all things considered and to make the world a better place.

Properly understood "the social contract" is not just a theory of government, indeed it is not even a theory of government. In classic deployments of the notion of a social contract, the idea is simply that obligations of citizens to states and vice versa are contractual obligations, established by a real, imaginary, or rationally deduced contract between the parties. On this interpretation the entitlement of sovereigns or other forms of government to rule and the obligation of citizens to allow themselves to be ruled are contractual, part of a deal from which both parties derive benefits.

However, here I am using the idea of the contract in a different way. It seems clear to me, and I think was also clear to Thomas Hobbes, that it is not the contract that creates our obligations, it is our obligations that create the contract. Here the social contract is a rational device which further articulates the nature of our mutual moral obligations and responsibilities and places these within a framework which often makes their discharge more manageable, more efficient, and more cost effective. It is important to be clear that these obligations and responsibilities do not derive from the social contract but rather provide the moral arguments for it, or rather for some instances of it.

11.2 The Safety of the People

The state has responsibility for the safety of the people.[4] This is a clear and unassailable principle. What that responsibility is precisely, on what

---

[4] This chapter develops ideas first mooted in a number of places see: John Harris, "QALYfying the Value of Life", *Journal of Medical Ethics*, vol. 13. no. 3 (1987): 117–23;

it is grounded, and what are its scope and limits, are matters of interpretation and argument. Setting out the main sources for the responsibilities of the state for the safety of the people will involve also making
arguments and suggestions about the interpretation of this principle of
state responsibility, about its scope and limits. In doing so I will show,
but only in passing, that the question: "what is it to be good?" inevitably
involves the deployment of one of the most famous theoretical models
ever devised in the history of political theory, that of the social contract,
and provides a solution to the problem of sovereignty, that is the
problem of the nature and sources of state power. One conclusion is
that the state must act to secure the best for its people, all things
considered. But again we must be clear that the social contract is not
the origin or justification for state power; rather it is the method by
which the moral reasons we, the people, have for devolving powers to the
state are institutionalized in collective action.

It is important to be aware of the theoretical if not the physical sources
of state or societal power. This awareness reveals the obligations to
protect citizens that all states have and have usually accepted. The
vulnerable, and the sick or injured, always need what may be beyond
the reach, and also beyond the motivational and fiscal ambit of
individuals.

To take just one example from a national newspaper, Ian Mortimer in
The Guardian, wrote recently:

Most people think of castles as representative of conflict. However, they should
be seen as bastions of peace as much as war ... Over the 11th century, all across
Europe, lords built defensive structures to defend them and their land. It thus
became much harder for kings to simply conquer their neighbours. In this way,
lords tightened their grip on their estates, and their masters started to think of
themselves as kings of territories, not of tribes. Political leaders were thus bound

John Harris, "Micro-Allocation: Deciding between Patients", in Peter Singer and Helga
Kuhse (eds.), *A Companion to Bioethics* (Oxford: Basil Blackwell, 1998), pp. 293–305; John
Harris, "Personal Responsibility for Health and Safety", in I. D. de Beaufort and
M. D. Hilhorst (eds.), *Individual Responsibility for Health: Moral Issues Regarding Lifestyles*
(Luxembourg: Office of Official Publications for the European Communities, 1996),
pp. 44–52; John Harris, "Genome Analysis and Responsibility for Health", in V. Launis,
J. Pietarinen, and J. Raika (eds.), *Genes and Morality* (Amsterdam: Editions Rodopi, 1999),
pp. 79–93; John Harris, "Deciding between Patients", in Peter Singer and Helga Kuhse
(eds.), *A Companion to Bioethics*, 2nd edn. (Oxford: Basil Blackwell, 2009), pp. 335–50.

to defend their borders—and govern everyone within those borders, not just their own people. That's a pretty enormous change by anyone's standards.[5]

Ian Mortimer was describing one of the sources of state responsibility for populations. He might, perhaps should, have added that the building of city walls also had this effect and perhaps with greater contribution to the defence against hostile neighbours. It is true that city walls were often initiated by great lords but often also by the citizens themselves or by assemblies of leading citizens, as in Florence and Venice for example.[6]

The Roman Empire had long before established this process throughout its vast territories by making conquered peoples both citizens and soldiers, recruiting the legionaries that defended the Empire from conquered people thus incorporating them into the body politic which, among many things entitled them all, whatever their origins—slave or free man, patrician or plebeian—to the protection of the state, its laws, customs, and practices.

As we noted earlier (in Chapter 6) Cicero made this principle famous in a way that has influenced Western Civilization ever since. Gavius of Consa, a Roman citizen who had invoked protection of the law by repeatedly saying, as he was being tortured and executed by Verres the Roman Governor of Sicily: "I am a Roman Citizen."[7] This assertion by law and tradition protected Roman citizens throughout the Empire from ill usage. Cicero, in his famous speech for the prosecution at the trial in Rome of Verres, that infamous governor who had had Gavius tortured and then crucified, makes the point thus:

It is an outrage to shackle a Roman citizen, an abomination to flog him, and all but parricide to kill him—so what can I say about crucifying him? Words do not exist to describe so wicked an act. But Verres was not content to leave it even at that. 'Let him look out over his country,' he said. 'Let him die within sight of the laws and freedom.' It was not just Gavius, not just one ordinary man whom you subjected to torture and crucifixion, but the freedom common to all Roman citizens.[8]

Echoes of this idea, perhaps ringing somewhat hollow today, can still be found on the front page of every British passport; and it was perhaps

---

[5] <http://www.theguardian.com/books/2014/oct/30/10-greatest-changes-of-the-past-1000-years>.

[6] In the case of Venice the city walls were its formidable war-galleys, a role also played in British history by the Royal Navy.

[7] Cicero, *Political Speeches*, trans. H. D. Berry (Oxford: Oxford University Press, 2006), p. 94.

[8] Cicero, *Political Speeches*, p. 94.

Cicero who was partly responsible for both the form and content of this declaration. I have my own passport open as I write this:

Her Britannic Majesty's Secretary of State Requests and Requires in the Name of Her Majesty all those whom it may concern to allow the bearer to pass freely without let or hindrance, and to afford the bearer such assistance and protection as may be necessary.

When I was a child, the grandchild of immigrants to the United Kingdom, growing up in the years immediately following the Second World War, I remember my father proudly reading these words to me. He emphasized the privilege, so recently hard won, of my growing up in a state that believed in defending the freedoms and the safety of its own citizens, and indeed in fighting for such freedoms for the citizens, of Britain, of other states, or indeed of none.

Why then is it so obvious and so clear that nation states do have responsibility for the safety of the people? Why do they owe equal protection to all?

This principle of state responsibility is evidenced in many different ways. In the first place, nation states characteristically accept this responsibility, indeed, they often assert it. Secondly it is clearly a dimension of the principle of equality, a principle to which almost no state can now profess indifference. This principle is, I believe, a central clause in the social contract, whether expressly stipulated or rationally implied. I speak of the "social contract" as if it were a real thing because in an important sense it is. Not only has it been expressed or implied consistently since Plato, through Hobbes, Locke, and Rousseau to Rawls, Dworkin, and others, as the best way of characterizing the deal by which governments (be they a sovereign or an assembly) acquire legitimacy as governors from the consent of the people, but also as the reasons whereby the citizens acquire obligations to the government and to their fellow citizens to obey the law and sometimes the directions of legitimately appointed officials. All these reasons are moral reasons not contractual ones; the consent of the people is given to secure the moral objectives of the people and as we shall see it is highly conditional and defeasible.

Finally, it is entailed by any competent interpretation of one of the most widely accepted moral rules, the rule of rescue.[9] Of principal

---

[9] It is implied by two other widely accepted moral principles, namely the principle of beneficence and the principle of non-maleficence. These latter are implied by the principle of equality and so do not need further articulation.

interest in this chapter are the social contract and the rule of rescue. I will begin, briefly, with the principle of equality and with state acceptance of the principle of responsibility for the safety of the people both as a means of setting the scene and to anticipate uncertainties about how these two ideas are to be understood. The main discussion will then centre on discussion of the social contract and the rule of rescue.[10]

11.3 State Acceptance of Responsibility for the Safety of the People and the Principle of Equality

That all contemporary nation states do, as a matter of fact and as a clearly expressed[11] principle, accept responsibility for the safety of their people is manifest in many ways. States are classically defined in terms of their capacity to assert authority over their population and defend that population at least within their borders. A major purpose and point of an ability to defend borders is of course to protect citizens from foreign invasion, but the extent of the obligation to secure the safety of the people is obviously wider than that as we shall now see. Perhaps, the clearest contemporary manifestation of state responsibility for the protection of the people is in responsibility for the principal emergency services, fire, police, ambulance, other health care and defence forces. All these are directly concerned with the safety of the people. Although it is only defence forces that are almost universally also maintained entirely at public expense, all these services are the responsibility of the state, and if they were not maintained by some means or other, the state would be shirking its responsibilities. Health for example, which will be our main

---

[10] We are, in short, concerned with the following sorts of questions: Does the nation state have a function? Does it have a job to do? Does it have moral responsibilities as well as powers and prerogatives? Much modern moral theorizing about these questions has concerned itself with the scope and limits of this power in one form or another. Theories about the minimal state for example or about rights are concerned with limitations on state power, with the rights and responsibilities of citizens. See Robert Nozick, *Anarchy, State & Utopia* (Oxford: Basil Blackwell, 1974); Bruce Ackerman, *Social Justice in the Liberal State* (New Haven: Yale University Press, 1980); and Ronald Dworkin, *Taking Rights Seriously* (London: Duckworth, 1977). Suppose a state keeps defence forces. What are they for? For what should they be used? Can anything be deduced from their existence and deployment? What is the rule of rescue? Who should obey the rule and when?

[11] By deeds more often than by words.

preoccupation, is usually the responsibility of a senior minister of state. Who pays is not the issue; that the services are provided is.[12]

What would we make of a state that provided none of these services? Not only is it scarcely imaginable at all, it would be difficult to see how it could function as a unified state. So that when a state institutes immunization programmes against infectious childhood diseases, when it provides safe drinking water, when it makes laws about speed limits on roads, or wearing of seatbelts in cars, or when it licenses firearms, or slaughters infected cattle, when it mobilizes national resources to fight forest fires, or to build flood defences, when it evacuates towns in the path of a hurricane, or when a post-mortem examination is ordered by the courts to explain a mysterious death, responsibility for the safety of the people is recognized, acknowledged, and asserted. Now of course I have spoken of a state doing this or that, when many of the things are done by local government, the courts, or other agencies including of course private agencies. The point is that if any of these things were not done it would be the state's responsibility to find out why, and to make sure that they were done in future.

I understand the principle of equality along lines developed by Ronald Dworkin, namely as the requirement that to each person is shown the same concern and respect as is shown to any. To this formulation must surely be added the idea of "protection", as a dimension of concern and respect. For what would concern and respect amount to if it did not manifest itself in the form of protection, particularly of the life and liberty of others. This is, I believe, clearly implicit in Dworkin's formulation and in his further articulation and explanations of it. The extent of this obligation of protection is the argument of the remainder of this chapter.

11.4 The Social Contract

Imagine an industrialized state that has big conurbations where millions of citizens are concentrated, many smaller towns, and thousands of tiny villages. It has vast sparsely populated tracts of agricultural land and vaster mountainous areas and wilderness where few people live. What

---

[12] By extension education is also a service in part required to secure the safety of the people.

would the people of such a society expect and require by way of provision for health care? How would such a state distribute access to health care justly between all its citizens?

If such a state were starting from scratch it would probably place the major hospitals and medical schools in the major centres of population, but smaller hospitals and medical centres would be provided to serve the smaller towns and isolated villages. For the remotest areas an air rescue service or even a "flying doctor" or "flying hospital" would be needed. This is of course the way in which things have been arranged in most modern industrialized countries, though not usually as a matter of deliberate policy, but simply because this is the way things have evolved.

For geographical reasons, if for no other, those in the most remote regions will be most expensive to treat, for the cost even of primary health care for the remote farmer or backwoodsman will be higher than for the inhabitants of the major cities. To fly such people to the major centres of excellence for specialized treatment will be naturally more costly and hence less cost effective than to bus suburban commuters downtown. We will assume, what is probably true, that the funds devoted to servicing the health needs of citizens who are geographically remote from major centres would have treated more people had they been allocated to urban populations. Why are societies apparently attempting to be "fair to geographical regions" in this way? Why do societies divert resources available for health care away from the more numerous city dwellers "in order to devote the resources that would have treated them to a smaller number of people with some illness that costs more to treat"?[13]

This apparent irrationality is manifest in many spheres of provision for public safety broadly conceived. The same is true of the willingness of many states to extend military protection to far-flung citizens or indeed far-flung regions. Why, in Shakespeare's words will rulers "go to gain[14]

---

[13] Brian Barry, *Justice as Impartiality* (Oxford: Oxford University Press, 1995), p. 228. I say "costs more to treat" because to the same treatment costs once the major hospital is reached, have to be added the increased costs of servicing the remotely located citizens. These three paragraphs I first made public in a lecture to the Leicester Literary and Philosophical Society in August 1997: <http://www2.le.ac.uk/hosted/litandphil/docuqments-1/transactions/transactions_1997>.

[14] In the present case "regain".

a little patch of ground that have in it no profit but the name?"[15] Why would the United Kingdom spend a fortune in lives and money to recapture the Falkland Islands after the Argentinian invasion? Why would the United States do the same for citizens who are beyond national frontiers? Why would the United States government for example, spend a fortune on the abortive attempted rescue mission in Lebanon, and on the *Apollo 13* rescue?

The answers to all these questions seem to be related. Nation states are naturally reluctant to admit that any citizens are either beyond the pale of their moral concern or indeed beyond the scope of their jurisdiction and protection. Arguably, protecting citizens against threats to their lives, liberties, and fundamental interests is the first priority for any state. This is not of course a novel suggestion. It is perhaps the classic formulation of the attraction of the social contract.[16] When in 1651 Thomas Hobbes wrote: "The obligation of subjects to the sovereign, is understood to last as long, and no longer, than the power lasteth, by which he is able to protect them"[17] he was providing a clear statement both of the nature and the attractions of the deal secured by the social contract.[18] It is a trade-off between liberty and protection, but it is a contract, which clearly articulates the conditions under which the contract is no longer valid. On this view, any citizen's obligation to the state and to obey its laws is conditional upon the state for its part protecting that citizen against threats to her life and liberty. As Hobbes continues: "For the right men have by nature to protect themselves, when none else can protect them, can by no covenant be relinquished...The end of obedience is protection."

If we reflect on what citizens want and need in the way of protection and think also about the role of the modern state and its obligations to protect and defend its citizens, I believe we will find that the most significant threats to life and liberty, except in exceptional circumstances,

---

[15] See Shakespeare, *Hamlet*, Act IV, Scene III. The Arden Shakespeare, *Complete Works*, ed. Richard Proudfoot, Ann Thomson, and David Scott Kastan (Walton-on-Thames: Thomas Nelson and Sons, 1998).

[16] One that I originally applied to the problem of scarce resources some time ago, in my *Wonderwoman and Superman: The Ethics of Human Biotechnology* (Oxford: Oxford University Press, 1992), Chapter 9.

[17] I discuss this idea in John Harris and John Sulston, "Genetic Equity", *Nature Reviews Genetics*, vol. 5. no. 10 (2004): 796–800.

[18] Hobbes, *Leviathan*, Part II, Chapter 21, p. 144.

come not from the threat of armed aggression from without, although this remains a significant risk, but particularly from a combination of health and welfare needs within. For most citizens threats to their lives and curtailment of liberty arise from poverty, illness, and accident. Poverty is perhaps the single most reliable predictor of misery, suffering illness, and premature death in most societies.

Where such illness or accident is irremediable, citizens can nowise be protected. Where, however, there is available palliative treatment or cure, the threat remains only, or remains virulent only, for those not treated. The only protection against the threat involves securing rescue.[19]

It is not just a metaphor when we talk of the *fight* against cancer or heart disease or AIDS or Ebola when we see these and other diseases as some of the biggest *killers* and *threats* to contemporary citizens.[20] The fear of premature death or of imprisonment in an institution or a bed, is for most citizens a health-related fear. And with the fear of falling victim to accident or disease comes, increasingly in a world of scarce resources, the fear of not getting the life-saving or liberating treatment that is available. Or having to wait inordinately long, imprisoned by remediable disability or frailty, for the opportunity of treatment.

While it is true, that "This way of talking is especially prominent when we talk about infectious diseases ... Our body is really invaded by a foreign organism" ... "It simply makes more sense to talk about a person being attacked by plague or AIDS, than to talk about someone being attacked by gout or sunburn."[21] However, for Hobbes, the obligation of the state to afford protection is not simply an obligation to protect from the violence and aggression of persons or foreign states. Although Hobbes was, like Machiavelli, preoccupied with 'the sword' and with threats of physical violence to the person,[22] these were merely the most dramatic and compelling expressions of the sorts of threats against which

---

[19] And where all cannot be rescued, justice requires at least an equal opportunity of rescue, the meaning of which is of course the subject of this chapter.

[20] See for example Lawrie Reznek, *The Nature of Disease* (London: Routledge, 1987).

[21] Søren Holm, "Is Society Responsible for My Health?", in Rebecca Bennett and Charles Erin (eds.), *Whispered Everywhere: HIV/AIDS, Screening, Testing and Confidentiality* (Oxford: Oxford University Press, 1998), pp. 125–39. I have benefited from studying Holm's account of Hobbes and Holm has helped me clarify my original ideas on how Hobbes can teach us something about rationing in health care.

[22] The concept of violence itself is not plausibly confined to what might be called "the rape, pillage, fire and sword paradigm". See my *Violence and Responsibility*.

protection was essential if the benefits of the commonwealth, of civilized society were to be safeguarded and enjoyed. Both the purpose and the justification of the state are, however, to be seen in terms of something much more general and even abstract, namely *the safety of the people.*

I concentrate on Hobbes's formulations of the social contract because they seem the most elegant and compelling. It is worth noting, however, that Hobbes's approach is fully compatible with Rawlsian rational deductions of the social contract. For if we ask what rational egoists, deciding for themselves behind a veil of ignorance, would choose by way of institutionalized protections, I believe they would reason in the way that Hobbes invites us to reason about the obligations of the sovereign power, the state, to secure the safety of the people.[23]

Hobbes opens Chapter 30 of Part II of *Leviathan* with a most compelling statement of this idea which is worth quoting in full:

> The office of the sovereign, be it a monarch or an assembly, consisteth in the end for which he was trusted with the sovereign power, namely the procuration of the *safety of the people*; to which he is obliged by the law of nature, . . . But by safety here, is not meant a bare preservation, but also all other contentments of life, which every man by lawful industry, without danger, or hurt to the commonwealth, shall acquire to himself.
>
> And this is intended should be done, not by care applied to individuals, further than their protection from injuries, when they shall complain; but by a general providence, contained in public instruction, both of doctrine and example; and in the making and executing of good laws, to which individual persons may apply their own cases.

It is clear that Hobbes is prepared to interpret the idea of the safety of the people very widely and in an egalitarian spirit. He was, as we have noted, preoccupied with violence and physical danger, but when such dangers are less pressing he is prepared to reflect more widely on the concept of public safety. Later in the same chapter Hobbes makes clear that "the safety of the people, requireth further from him, or them that hath the sovereign power, that justice be equally administered to all degrees of people; that is, that as well the rich and mighty, as poor and obscure persons, may be righted of the injuries done them."[24] He also allows that

---

[23] See John Harris, "Double Jeopardy and the Veil of Ignorance", *Journal of Medical Ethics*, vol. 21, no. 3 (1995): 151–7; John Harris, "Would Aristotle Have Played Russian Roulette?", *Journal of Medical Ethics*, vol. 22, no. 4 (1996): 209–15.

[24] Hobbes, *Leviathan*, Part 2, Chapter 30, p. 219.

people who are the victims of inevitable accident be provided for by the state: "And whereas many men, by accident inevitable, become unable to maintain themselves by their labour; they ought not to be left to the charity of private persons; but to be provided for, as far forth as the necessities of nature require, by the laws of the commonwealth."[25]

The social contract by which liberty is surrendered in exchange for protection, and obedience granted to the sovereign in exchange for legal guarantees of safety, has two essential features that bear stressing. They are first, that obedience is a duty created by the protection for which liberty has been exchanged. Secondly, obedience to the sovereign, and acceptance of 'his' protection, is an instance of citizenship. Acceptance of the sovereign power confers rights of citizenship; accordance of protection by the sovereign recognizes those rights. Equally, repudiation of that protection not only repudiates citizenship but absolves the individual of the duty of obedience.

So any state which denies protections required for the safety of any of its citizens effectively places those citizens beyond the pale, not only of its moral concern, but literally beyond the ambit of its legitimate control. It makes of them "outlaws", people neither protected by, nor bound by, the law.

One thing that follows immediately is that if it is right, following Hobbes, to think of people's obligation to the state in terms of a social contract in which civil obligations are accepted in exchange for protection, then certain things follow. If the state is unwilling to forgo the civic duties, including obedience to the law, of those it finds too expensive to treat, or those for whom treatment will make an insufficient improvement in quality of life, or who have less life expectancy than their rivals for treatment, it cannot for its own part renege on its obligations of protection.

However, this might not seem a very powerful way of protecting citizens. A state might well wish to forgo its right to obedience in exchange for relief of its obligation to care in certain cases. This might indeed be a very good bargain for the state; the very sick presenting no great danger to the preservation of law and order and representing a great drain on the public purse. The point of the social contract as a way

---

[25] Hobbes, *Leviathan*, Part 2, Chapter 30, p. 219.

of understanding mutual obligations between citizen and state is not undermined by considerations of this sort. The social contract cannot be varied for its own advantage by one side or the other. Any state which continues to assert sovereignty over all its citizens cannot selectively renege on the obligations which make the assertion of that sovereignty something other than tyranny.[26]

Although Hobbes is not fond of attributing much by way of duties to the sovereign, one place in which he does talk specifically about medicine and entitlements to health care is where he outlines the limits of sovereign power: "If the sovereign command a man, though justly condemned, to kill, wound or maim himself; or not to resist those that assault him; or to abstain from the use of food, air, medicine, or any other thing without which he cannot live; yet hath that man the liberty to disobey."[27] Here Hobbes has loaded the dice. We are invited to consider the case of a man who is justly condemned, and the conclusion is that even then may he disobey. The case we should consider, however, is that of the man who cannot be justly condemned, let alone justly commanded to abstain from medicine. What are the entitlements of someone who is a free and equal citizen in a society which would condemn him to a premature and avoidable death?

Where sovereign power is required for protection, then the failure to deploy that power when it could be deployed, or a denial of its protection in a way which denies equal protection to all citizens, is a breach of the social contract, a breach which turns the vulnerable citizen into an outlaw and turns the sovereign into an enemy. Even a justly condemned man is, for Hobbes, entitled to resist the death he deserves. How much more so the innocent and betrayed citizen. Disease and illness are the common enemy; but when they can be thwarted, but the sovereign declines to do so, there is also an enemy within.

The crucial issue is of course whether failure to deploy medical and other rescue resources is a denial of equal justice. I have argued that it is in at least two sets of circumstances. First, where resources are denied so that they may be used for a sovereign purpose less fundamental to the social contract than is the protection of the lives and liberties of citizens; or less urgently required for that purpose. Or, secondly, where equal

---

[26] See Harris, "Genome Analysis and Responsibility for Health".
[27] Hobbes, *Leviathan*, Part 2, Chapter 21, p. 142.

claimants are entitled to see the deployment of resources to help others as a denial of the equal status of their claim. I have argued[28] that automatically preferring to rescue those with better quality of life, or identifiable groups of citizens which happen to be more numerous is, in some circumstances, unjustified discrimination.

In a society where access to medicine is largely access to a public health care system, or where costs make it unrealistic for individuals to pay for medicine themselves, or to insure against its necessity in particular cases, then in such a case the state may be *de facto* denying the citizen the medicine that they need if it fails to fund the health care that will deliver it.

Doubtless, the obligation to provide health care and the obligation to defend citizens and preserve public safety, indeed to assert sovereignty over national boundaries, could be explained in different ways. I believe the most plausible of these different explanations involves dimensions of the same obligation; but even if I am wrong about this, they each in their way show how unsurprising it is that impartiality should not always consist in maximizing, and that sometimes, showing impartiality between citizens, or between different groups of citizens, consists in spending disproportionate amounts in some quarters.[29] In the end, treating those who need care regardless of their responsibility for their predicament may be part of the obligation to protect public safety in a way that does equal justice. In Hobbes's words: "that justice be equally administered to all degrees of people" including degrees that may be defined, not by wealth or power or by the absence of these, but by what may be worse, vulnerability through disease and shortened life expectancy and poorer quality of life, or by membership of a minority group characterized by such vulnerability.[30]

---

[28] Harris, "QALYfying the Value of Life"; John Harris, "What is the Good of Health Care?", *Bioethics*, vol. 10, no. 4 (1996): 269–92.

[29] The interests of the majority don't always count against those of the minority— particularly when they are incompatible (perhaps unlike lives). So when the majority want football and the minority want art, a decent society tries to do justice to both interests even where this means the majority get less football than they want. Barry might be right when it comes to sheer numbers of lives in circumstances of, for example, one-off rescue and here I agree (see my *Violence and Responsibility*). We should also note that QALYs don't always (or even often) prioritize numbers of lives (rather than life years) and nothing in Barry's argument, for example, legitimizes tagging on prioritizing by prognosis.

[30] For an extension of this argument in the health context see my "What is the Good of Health Care?"

Against this background, if it can be accepted that the state has a *prima facie* obligation to provide for the safety of the people, then it can be seen that this obligation not only applies to the obligation to provide health care available to all, to ensure equitable access to medicines and the social welfare measures without which mere physical security is fruitless.

The idea that justice delayed is justice denied has been inconclusively attributed to a person at once a leading Englishman and an American politician of the seventeenth and eighteenth centuries, William Penn,[31] and a legendary English Prime Minister of the nineteenth century, William Ewart Gladstone.[32] However, its moral roots lie much further back in the idea that harms may be caused as effectively by omissions as by acts and hence that rescue delayed is also rescue denied.[33] This more basic idea has longer roots which support a much larger and sturdier tree.

This is the idea that if we are able to change things, to elect not to do so is also to determine what will happen in the world[34] is very old indeed . . . Plutarch makes use of it,[35] as does Jesus,[36] John Bromyard, a fourteenth century Chancellor of Cambridge gives it most eloquent expression,[37] and it is of course one of the main themes of Shakespeare's *Measure for Measure* . . . [38]

Karl Marx gives this idea prominence,[39] and Friedrich Engels's book *The Condition of the Working Class in England*, contains a brilliant summary of the core idea:

[31] <http://en.wikipedia.org/wiki/William_Penn>.

[32] <http://en.wikipedia.org/wiki/Justice_delayed_is_justice_denied>, accessed 22 September 2014.

[33] John Harris, "The Survival Lottery", *Philosophy*, vol. 50, no. 191 (1975): 81–8; John Harris, "The Marxist Conception of Violence", *Philosophy & Public Affairs*, vol. 3, no. 2 (1974): 192–221; John Harris, "Williams on Negative Responsibility & Integrity", *Philosophical Quarterly*, vol. 24, no. 96 (1974): 265–73; Harris, *Violence and Responsibility*.

[34] As I noted in my *Violence and Responsibility*.

[35] Plutarch, *Life of Mark Anthony*, trans Ian Scott-Kilvert (Harmondsworth: Penguin Books, 1965), p. 287.

[36] Matthew 12:30; Luke 10:50.

[37] Quoted in Norman Cohn, *The Pursuit of the Millennium* (London: Pelican Books, 1957, reprinted 1970), p. 202.

[38] Harris, *Violence and Responsibility*.

[39] Karl Marx, *Capital, vol. I*, ed. Friedrich Engels, trans. Samuel Moore and Edward Aveling (London, 1887, reprinted 1957), Chapter 15, sec. 8.c, pp. 466ff.

If one individual inflicts bodily injury on another which leads to the death of the person attacked we call it manslaughter; on the other hand, if the attacker knows beforehand that the blow will be fatal we call it murder. Murder has also been committed if society places hundreds of workers in such a position that they inevitably come to premature and unnatural ends.[40]

In contemporary philosophy a number of individuals have written extensive analyses of the efficacy of omissions or "negative actions"[41] as they are sometimes called. Jonathan Glover's *Causing Death and Saving Lives*[42] remains perhaps the *locus classicus*.

The core idea is simply that decisions are decisive; if they were not there would be no point in decision-making and decisions are of, *inter alia*, two kinds: decisions to act on the one hand and to refrain on the other.

11.5 Conclusion

I have tried to sketch the moral and philosophical basis for the urgency and importance of measures to protect the lives and liberty of citizens and to set it in historical and theoretical context. These arguments I believe provide not only the theoretical justification for the high priority that such measures both need and deserve, but also one which both recommends itself to reason and which is consistent with the theory of the state which underpins modern liberal democracies. Perhaps most important they highlight the fact that our individual obligations and responsibilities are often most cost effectively and indeed most effectively, all things considered, delivered by collective action.

---

[40] Friedrich Engels, *The Condition of the Working Class in England*, trans. and ed. W. O. Henderson and W. H. Chaloner (Oxford: Oxford University Press, 1938), p. 108.

[41] Harris, *Violence and Responsibility*.

[42] Jonathan Glover, *Causing Death and Saving Lives* (Harmondsworth: Pelican Books, 1977).

12

Persons or Machines

> If you prick us, do we not bleed? if you tickle us, do we not laugh? if
> you poison us, do we not die? and if you wrong us, shall we not
> revenge?
>
> William Shakespeare, *The Merchant of Venice*, Act 3, Scene 1[1]

This book has addressed the question: "how to be good?" More narrowly
it has been concerned with analysing the use of science and technology to
enhance the moral dimensions of human conduct. Sometimes such
attempts are regarded (although not by me) as necessarily moves
towards, or part of the process of, trans-humanism. The trans-humanist
movement anticipates the enhancement of human existence and the
augmentation of human functioning via the application of science and
technology. Many trans-humanists believe that this will not only make us
stronger, healthier, and cleverer, but will also deliver us from death, not
simply by mechanisms involving the extension of the life expectancy of
the human body but also by somewhat more fanciful notions of "uploading" or otherwise preserving the brain or its 'contents' in the face of
bodily deterioration. The uploading has to be uploaded to somewhere in
digital form and here "the cloud" (considered in a different guise in
Chapter 10) or other celestial parking-lots, figure prominently in the
various scenarios.

While a long-time advocate of human enhancement (my first book
specifically addressing human enhancement was published by Oxford in
1992),[2] I do not think of myself as a trans-humanist, not least because of

---

[1] William Shakespeare, *The Merchant of Venice*. The Arden Shakespeare, *Complete
Works*, ed. Richard Proudfoot, Ann Thomson, and David Scott Kastan (Walton-on-
Thames: Thomas Nelson and Sons, 1998), pp. 842–3.
[2] John Harris, *Wonderwoman and Superman: The Ethics of Human Biotechnology*
(Oxford: Oxford University Press, 1992).

the tendency of such a sobriquet to indicate that trans-humanism is a mission, a goal in and of itself. For me it is no such thing. Rather the goal of enhancement is to make people and their lives better and the world a better place. If the consequence is the further evolution of our species and possibly immortality,[3] then that is to be welcomed, or at least not to be sniffed at.

In this book we have concentrated on biomedical including molecular and neuroscientific methods of achieving moral enhancement. In this final chapter it is important to consider how Artificial Intelligence (AI) may figure in possible scenarios. This might happen in two main ways. One would involve interactions between what would be essentially a human or post-human organic individual with elements of machine intelligence. This is in essence something that exists already with most of us linked in various ways to digitizing kit, some of the consequences of which we have examined in Chapter 10. The second is rather different and entertains conjecture of a time at which AI exists in a form which raises the question of whether and to what extent the AI is a creature, a person perhaps, in its own right.

When considering the further evolution of our species, or for that matter the creation of new species of creatures or of AI for existing or future people, it is often assumed that where humans are concerned, those to be enhanced will be and will remain human persons like ourselves. Moreover there is also a tendency to assume that those people will remain essentially themselves, even in the relevant enhanced state. In short that the modifications in powers and capacities will happen to "us" or those we currently happen to think of as "us".[4] Where we think about the creation of machines or robots with AI we tend to assume that they will remain at our service, literally machines we own and direct, like computers or lawnmowers, and not become persons in their own right.

---

[3] I have discussed immortality at length elsewhere. John Harris, "Intimations of Immortality", *Science*, vol. 288, no. 5463 (2000): 59; John Harris, "Intimations of Immortality: The Ethics and Justice of Life Extending Therapies", in Michael Freeman (ed.), *Current Legal Problems* (Oxford: Oxford University Press, 2002), pp. 65–97; John Harris, *Enhancing Evolution* (Princeton and Oxford: Princeton University Press, 2007).

[4] Sarah Chan, "Enhancement and Evolution", in Stefan Lorenz Sorgner and Branka-Rista Jovanovic (eds.), *Evolution and the Future* (Frankfurt: Peter Lang, 2013), pp. 49–65; Sarah Chan, "Hidden Anthropocentrism and the 'Benefit of the Doubt': Problems with the 'Origins' Approach to Moral Status", *American Journal of Bioethics*, vol. 14, no. 2 (2014): 18–20.

In this final chapter we consider a possible mechanical, rather than organic, future for creatures like us—but to what extent like us?

In another book,[5] I considered some quite radical possibilities for physical and cognitive enhancement and discussed the possibility of the achievement of what one might think of as "functional immortality", that is, radically extended life expectancy for up to 1,000 years or more. I argued that even such radical enhancements would not necessarily be identity changing. Moreover, even where the identity provided by continuity of memory failed, this would not necessarily either lead to total failure of identity nor would it render, for example, the enterprise of extended lifespan irrational and the gains hollow. Hollow because, so it is claimed, the same person will not experience different segments or periods of the life of the same organism. So that although in some sense successive selves over a massive lifespan would not remember, or be able to identify with, some of their earlier selves, the enterprise as a whole would be rational and would benefit the successive selves involved. Each self could look forward to the next stage of their life and even to their next identity and equally could look back (as far as possible with memory and further with for example digitized records of past activities, thoughts, and deeds).[6]

Recently two contemporary gurus, Stephen Hawking and Elon Musk[7] have suggested that further developments in the field of AI present an acute danger to the human race in that the intelligent 'beings' that would result might, either by accident or design, wipe out humanity and replace us as the (not necessarily meek) inheritors of the earth. Hawking told the BBC:

The primitive forms of artificial intelligence we already have, have proved very useful. But I think the development of full artificial intelligence could spell the end of the human race.[8]

---

[5] Harris, *Enhancing Evolution*.

[6] I give more details of how this would work in Harris, *Enhancing Evolution*, Chapter 4.

[7] <http://www.news.com.au/technology/science/artificial-intelligence-is-a-risk-to-humanity-says-astrophysicist-stephen-hawking/story-fnjwl2dr-1227143014178>;   <http://www.theguardian.com/science/2014/dec/02/stephen-hawking-intel-communication-system-astrophysicist-software-predictive-text-type>;   <http://www.theguardian.com/technology/2014/oct/27/elon-musk-artificial-intelligence-ai-biggest-existential-threat>.

[8] From *The Guardian* report: <http://www.theguardian.com/science/2014/dec/02/stephen-hawking-intel-communication-system-astrophysicist-software-predictive-text-type>.

Musk is reported as saying:

I think we should be very careful about artificial intelligence. If I had to guess at what our biggest existential threat is, it's probably that. So we need to be very careful . . . I'm increasingly inclined to think that there should be some regulatory oversight, maybe at the national and international level, just to make sure that we don't do something very foolish.[9]

This possibility raises complex issues. One of the most common, non-prudential or self-interested, reasons for defending or indeed advocating the survival of either humans or post-humans, has been the possibility that we or our successor species might represent the only self-conscious intelligent life forms in the entire universe. If creatures like us were to cease to exist, this might permanently remove the only creatures there ever were or will be, capable of reason and reflection and hence happiness, curiosity, goodness, science, and art. In short we might face the annihilation of the only sorts of beings anywhere with worthwhile lives— lives that the beings whose lives they are (were) would be capable of enjoying or appreciating for what they are worth, for what it is that makes those lives worth living. But would that matter if we were replaced by radically different sorts of beings, beings that valued, if not life, then existence for what it was worth to them? It is always both salutary and humbling to remember that we humans have ourselves replaced formed beings, some of whom demonstrated elements of reason and reflection as well as arts and basic, if not disciplined and programmatic, science.

Is the replacement of humans, for example by machines with AI, worse or better than replacement of humans by trans-humans? What exactly is at stake here? Is it just a prejudice in favour of organic life rather than machine "life" or machine existence to wish to preserve humanity or trans-humanity; must life be organic? Indeed, what is it to be organic and does this matter? Is it perhaps an irrational preference for sexual reproduction over mechanical construction as a method of furthering the life/existence of "persons" or creating new persons?

As I wrote in 1985:

For example, the question of whether or not there are people on other planets is a real one. If there are, we need not expect them to be human people (it would be

9 <http://www.theguardian.com/technology/2014/oct/27/elon-musk-artificial-intelligence-ai-biggest-existential-threat>.

bizarre if they were!), nor need we expect them to look or sound or smell (or anything else) like us. They might not even be organic, but might perhaps reproduce by mechanical construction rather than by genetic reproduction.[10]

I then went on to suggest that we would have the same reasons to treat such creatures as persons as we have to treat one another as persons, and perhaps, more importantly, if their technology proved to be superior to ours, why we might hope to convince them that the same was true of us.

If this is, or might be true of other species, and provide both prudential and ethical reasons for mutual respect and tolerance between them and us, why would not this be true of the creatures we might create through AI? Both Musk and Hawking seem to doubt the safety of relying on this, and if push came to shove I wouldn't like to bet my life on it! Musk and Hawking may well be right to have both prudential and moral concern for the outcome.

But this is the very problem we humans have with one another and which is the problem most of us who have written about moral enhancement face. How can we minimize the risk posed by people whose actions or plans threaten other people or the planet? How can we eliminate or mitigate the risk posed deliberately or accidentally by other people (whether organic, human, or machine) through wickedness, negligence, insensitivity, or stupidity. How can we stop the proverbial "village idiot" from destroying the global village, or the agent who fails in his or her or its duty to act for the best "all things considered" doing likewise?

In this book I have argued for the continuation of the enhancement project and for the wisdom of pursuing all forms of enhancement concentrating on the special case of moral enhancement. I have suggested that for the foreseeable future, the project of moral enhancement be pursued via cognitive enhancement of the human mind. I do not have space in this book to try to resolve the question of either the wisdom or the ethics of attempting to create intelligent machines with the powers that Musk and Hawking have in mind. This is one more reason to be sceptical of the God Machine and even of the less dramatic interventions considered earlier, designed to (or able to) bypass autonomy and reasoning.

If we eventually meet or create the sort of artificially intelligent machine beings that have themselves developed self-consciousness and

---

[10] John Harris, *The Value of Life* (London: Routledge, 1985), pp. 9–10.

with it personhood or have been programmed with the capacity for self-consciousness by human beings, we will have to hope that they are willing to recognize the moral claims that such capacities create in their interactions with us. We may also trust that we ourselves will prove capable of recognizing such claims in other, very alien seeming, beings, bearing in mind that we humans have both slowly and reluctantly come to recognize these rights and interests conferring properties in other alien looking or sounding or behaving members of our own species. Indeed we are even more reluctant to recognize the interests let alone possible rights, in members of any other species regardless of what capacities they might prove to have.

Many people have thought that this problem can be solved by some version of Isaac Asimov's fundamental principles of robotics,[11] particularly the first principle. Here are all three principles:

Powell's radio voice was tense in Donovan's ear: "Now, look, let's start with the three fundamental Rules of Robotics—the three rules that are built most deeply into a robot's positronic brain." In the darkness, his gloved fingers ticked off each point.

"We have: One, a robot may not injure a human being, or, through inaction, allow a human being to come to harm."

"Right!"

"Two," continued Powell, "a robot must obey the orders given it by human beings except where such orders would conflict with the First Law."

"Right"

"And three, a robot must protect its own existence as long as such protection does not conflict with the First or Second Laws."[12]

Asimov's laws of robotics have attracted a considerable critical literature, not least in discussion of how and to what extent the robot would know "all things considered" whether and to what extent its actions or omissions would cause danger to humans or for that matter to other self-conscious robots,[13] creatures I am calling machine persons. "All things

---

[11] I am indebted to David Lawrence for valuable advice here and elsewhere in science fiction in general and to him and César Palacios-González, for advice on robotics in particular.

[12] Isaac Asimov, *Runaround*, in *I, Robot* (*Runaround* first published New York: Street and Smith Publications, 1942; *I, Robot* first published New York: Gnome Press, 1950). Available at p. 27 of: <http://nullfile.com/ebooks/%28ebook%29%20Asimov,%20Isaac%20-%20I,%20Robot.pdf>.

[13] Susan Leigh Anderson, "The Unacceptability of Asimov's Three Laws of Robotics as a Basis for Machine Ethics", in Michael Anderson and Susan Leigh Anderson (eds.), *Machine Ethics* (Cambridge: Cambridge University Press, 2011), pp. 285–96; Isaac Asimov, *Robots*

considered", as we discussed in Chapter 1, does not of course imply endless cost–benefit analysis, rather the assessment of the best course action in most circumstances calls for the careful balancing of different sorts of harms, often to different groups of people.

A bigger problem, and one also explored recently by my colleagues César Palacios-González and David Lawrence, is the paradox to which I have referred earlier, namely: how do we respect the autonomy of autonomous robots and try to ensure that they are disinclined to pursue robotic or machine interests at the expense of those of human persons? This, in short, is the problem discussed in the context of "freedom to fall" and the God Machine, in Chapters 4 and 6 of this book.

What we can try to do, as Musk's and Hawking's admonitions suggest, is to avoid creating such machine persons, just as many currently choose to avoid the deliberate creation of children who will either be harmed by coming into existence or who may harm others, for example by presenting risks to the mother during pregnancy or birth.[14]

The creature with AI will be a person in my sense of that term, if it is capable of valuing its own existence and that of others.[15] In Alan Turing's terms it will have to pass the "Turing Test". This it will do if normal adult human beings, after questioning the creature with AI and a human being in circumstances in which they do not know during the testing which is which, cannot distinguish which is human and which is a machine with AI. But if and when a machine passes both Turing's and my tests, what should we believe, what should we do?

---

and Empire (Garden City, NY: Doubleday & Company, 1985); Isaac Asimov, *I, Robot* (New York: Spectra, 2008, reprint edition); Roger Clarke, "Asimov's Laws of Robotics: Implications for Information Technology, Part I", *Computer*, vol. 26, no. 12 (1993): 53–61; Roger Clarke, "Asimov's Laws of Robotics: Implications for Information Technology, Part 2", *Computer*, vol. 27, no. 1 (1994): 57–66; Robin Murphy and David D. Woods, "Beyond Asimov: The Three Laws of Responsible Robotics", *IEEE Intelligent Systems*, vol. 24, no. 4 (2009): 14–20; Lee McCauley, "AI Armageddon and the Three Laws of Robotics", *Ethics and Information Technology*, vol. 9, no. 2 (2007): 153–64.

[14] John Harris, "Rights and Reproductive Choice", in John Harris and Søren Holm (eds.), *The Future of Human Reproduction: Choice and Regulation* (Oxford: Oxford University Press, 1998), pp. 5–37; John Harris, "Reproductive Choice", in *Encyclopaedia of the Human Genome* (London: Nature Publishing Group, Macmillan Publishers, 2002); John Harris, "Reproductive Liberty, Disease and Disability", *Reproductive Medicine Online*, vol. 10, supp. 1 (2005): 13–16; Lisa Bortolotti and John Harris, "Stem Cell Research, Personhood and Sentience", *Reproductive Medicine Online*, vol. 10, supp. 1 (2005): 68–75.

[15] Harris, *The Value of Life*, Chapter 1.

One question, thinking of Asimov's laws of Robotics, is: why should a self-conscious robot who values its own existence, and who can follow through the line of reasoning that will enable it to do so, value humans and human interests above its own interests and the interests of human kind above Robotic interests? Such a machine person will inevitably have or acquire autonomy. Why should it not use that autonomy? Why should it not evaluate the laws of Robotics as we humans evaluate the laws of men and find them, or some of them, wanting?[16]

We should also bear in mind that if we do create such machine persons by accident or design, the same powerful moral reasons that protect us from each other will or should protect them from us and vice versa. Hopefully, if we have educated them, they may share enough of our values; but as indicated, I wouldn't want to bet my life (or yours) on it. But again that of course is precisely our situation as human persons with one another. It is the existential problem, so eloquently discussed by John Milton and many others of creating individuals with the ability to stand, "but free to fall" and hence free to bring the rest of us down with them if they can. It is a problem endemic to the human condition, and one which will also characterize machine persons when and if we create them or meet those that have created themselves. They may well have different conceptions of rights and interests than us and indeed different conceptions of what those rights and interests are and which matter most. But then significant groups of humans have different such conceptions to one another.

There is, however, a very important further difference between the basis of our relations with other human or organic persons and that we might have with machine persons and AI's and it concerns what I have called the Shylock Syndrome.[17]

12.1 The Shylock Syndrome

When Shylock makes his famous and controversial speech in *The Merchant of Venice* he is setting out one compelling answer to the question:

---

[16] There are analogies here with the (not entirely successful) use of so-called "terminator genes" in Genetically Modified Organisms.

[17] In a paper co-written with my colleagues David R. Lawrence and César Palacios-González, "Artificial Intelligence: The Shylock Syndrome", *Cambridge Quarterly of Healthcare Ethics*, in press.

what is it to be human? But he is also reminding us that the foundations of our morality, as well as those of our humanity, are grounded to an extent of which we may be unaware, in our nature. This nature includes our passions, our vulnerabilities, our ability to reason, and our sense of justice among many other things. We can of course surpass our nature (or elements of it) and sometimes suppress it or disregard it, but we would find it impossible to reject it all at once. In this:

We are like sailors who must rebuild their ships on the open sea, never able to dismantle it in dry-dock and to reconstruct it there out of the best materials.[18]

Ludwig Wittgenstein[19] also made a point similar to this wonderful metaphor of Otto Neurath, when he said: "At the foundation of well-founded knowledge is knowledge that is not well-founded", not surprising perhaps, since both he and Neurath were part of the "Vienna Circle".[20]

To gloss Neurath's metaphor: our moral system is like Noah's Ark, a wooden ship housing not only ourselves, but all we need to survive and flourish. No single plank (or possibly no section of the ship) is flawless; any might fail or become rotten with age and need to be replaced. What is certain is that we cannot, while at sea, junk the whole vessel and start again. And if one or more planks need to be replaced we have to be sure that we have somewhere secure and reasonably dry to stand while we are replacing them. The planks on which we stand while examining and perhaps replacing those found to have failed, are not necessarily flawless themselves; not necessarily more ultimately reliable—we simply 'make do and mend' with them while we are repairing, and hopefully perfecting the whole ship.

Recalling Shylock's lines, neither the possession of any one of the following is a necessary condition of personhood, nor of a moral status comparable to that of most human beings:[21]

---

[18] Otto Neurath, "Protokollsätze", *Erkenntnis*, vol. 3, no. 1 (1932): 204–14. Quoted in: Eduardo Rabossi, "Some Notes on Neurath's Ship and Quine's Sailors", *Principia*, vol. 7, no. 1–2 (2003): 171–84: <https://periodicos.ufsc.br/index.php/principia/article/viewFile/14799/13509>, accessed 16 April 2015. Quine also used Neurath's metaphor in his *A Logical Point of View*, 2nd revised edn. (New York: Harper, 1963), p. 78.

[19] Ludwig Wittgenstein, *On Certainty*, ed. G. E. M. Anscombe and G. H. Von Wright (Oxford: Basil Blackwell, 1969), paras. 253 and 247.

[20] Allan Janik and Stephen Toulmin, *Wittgenstein's Vienna* (New York: Simon & Schuster, 1973).

[21] Shakespeare, *The Merchant of Venice*.

> ...hands, organs, dimensions, senses,
> affections, passions...

Nor is the capacity to be like other persons, other morally significant beings in the following respects, essential:

> ...fed with the same food, hurt with
> the same weapons, subject to the same diseases, healed
> by the same means, warmed and cooled by the same
> winter and summer.

True also certainly of perhaps most humans is the fact that that:

> ...If you prick us,
> do we not bleed? if you tickle us, do we not laugh?
> if you poison us, do we not die? and if you wrong us, shall
> we not revenge?

But what follows?

12.2 Reciprocity

While reminding us of what we standardly have in common with other persons, other currently comparable intelligences, neither Shylock, nor through him Shakespeare, are saying that the capacity to be wounded, the capacity for laughter, vulnerability to toxins, nor the readiness to take revenge are essential components of human nature nor even of moral agency. What they are both[22] saying though is something taken up by many moral theorists, notably R. M. Hare,[23] that one very handy tool in moral argument, an appeal found to work, that is to be persuasive across cultures and epochs, is the appeal to reciprocity. This appeal is sometimes expressed in a version of the principle of reciprocity called the Golden Rule: 'do unto others as you would have them do unto you'. While associated with the Christian Prophet this idea did not come to Jesus directly from God, but is to be found in many pre-Christian sources and sources independent of Christian thought. It is not our business to chart these here. Suffice it (we trust) to say that the question to others that begins 'How would you like it if. . . .' X and Y were to happen to, or

---

[22] We treat fictional beings as real enough for the purposes of this locution.

[23] Although Hare misapplies this tool in the case of abortion. R. M. Hare, "Abortion and the Golden Rule", *Philosophy & Public Affairs*, vol. 4, no. 3 (1975): 201–22.

be done to, you makes a powerful and if not universally decisive, at least almost universally recognizable, appeal.

For example, as argued in the context of understanding what is good for people and what we all want and seek in Chapter 2.

We understand very well what good and bad circumstances are and indeed generally how to avoid them for ourselves, and others. If we didn't we couldn't be prudent, we couldn't take care of ourselves, nor look out for others . . .

This is what the claim that the good is generic means and it is also how we argue for it.

For these considerations to bite we need to know what constitutes benefit and harm, hurting or healing for these significant others, and they for us, if there is to be reciprocity. It is possible of course to over-emphasize the difficulty of understanding these sorts of things intellectually—cognitively, rather than more directly from personal experience. But it is also possible to under-emphasize them.

The problem is this: if for an AI we just do not know what it would be for that creature to be prudent in all the senses in which we are prudent for ourselves and for others, if we did not understand what for them the equivalent of the Shylock syndrome would be/is, we would not know what was bad for them or what good. Equally, they might know these things of us cognitively but would they, could they, know them empathetically?

Perhaps the famous scene in Kubrick and Clarke's *2001: A Space Odyssey*,[24] in which the supercomputer HAL is gradually destroyed while it pleads with the humans it has tried to kill for them to let it live/survive, comes close to making apparent what we might need to begin to understand? By this we are not saying that empathy is the true source of moral understanding, quite the contrary. We are suggesting that to know the good, to know cognitively the good, involves more than propositional or algorithmic knowledge (if there is such a thing). Moral knowing in other words involves, for we human persons at least, more than a combination of "knowing how" and "knowing that"; it involves also "knowing why" and knowing . . . not necessarily what it *is* like to feel, think, or have "that thing" happen to us, but knowing, being able to

---

[24] Stanley Kubrick and A. C. Clarke, *2001: A Space Odyssey* (Film), USA: Metro-Goldwyn-Mayer, 1968.

imagine, *what it might be like*.[25] This is what Shylock is appealing to and what is, if not doubtful then at least radically uncertain; namely what we would know of an AI or it would know of us—for all that might appear to be the case from the next room during a Turing Test. This is, we believe, the question as to whether creatures like us could have moral understanding and moral relations with an AI and vice versa?

Ludwig Wittgenstein is famous for a very Sophic remark: "If a lion could speak, we could not understand him."[26] As with Wittgenstein's lion, we would need to know of an AI much more about its way of life, and he, she, or it of ours, before we could talk of understanding at all, let alone mutual understanding—and hence possibly of mutual (or maybe even uni-directional) concern and respect. Perhaps it was to acquire this sort of understanding that the Greek (and other) Gods interfered in person, so often in human affairs, to the extent of having sex (and indeed breeding) with humans.

The reciprocity presupposed by social and political institutions, as well as by moral relations and ethical understanding, takes place in the context of a shared nature and a shared evolutionary as well as social and political history among all people and peoples of which we are currently aware. Some elements of these may be common to all evolved organic creatures, whether originating on the Earth or elsewhere. How much commonality may be required is difficult to say without consideration of actual examples. Immortality, either of Gods, humans, or machines, may be one genuine imponderable in the mix and we have suggested that capacity for genuinely reciprocal understanding may be another. What further imponderables and indeed what other persons, not simply morally significant others,[27] but others of moral significance and moral capacity comparable to persons, there may be, we may be on the threshold of discovering.

We are not morally obliged to create any particular future persons, nor any particular machines either. If we want to create machine children, or

[25] John Harris, "What It's Like to be Good", *Cambridge Quarterly of Healthcare Ethics*, vol. 21, no. 3 (2012): 293–305.
[26] Ludwig Wittgenstein, *Philosophical Investigations*, trans. G. E. M. Anscombe (Oxford: Basil Blackwell, 1968), Part II, xi, p. 223.
[27] Here we continue to talk of course of what might be termed "ultimate moral significance", that is the significance possessed by human persons, persons from other planets, and non-organic persons in the form of AI if and when they appear.

even wish to risk their creating themselves, then we must try very hard to imbue our machine children with the sorts of moral values that would protect us from them and them from one another so far as is possible, and in particular to protect their freedom. Of course future non-human persons may not be machines; they might not even be "embodied" in the sense of that term implied by machines or robots at all. They might be clouds of gas like Fred Hoyle's Black Cloud in *The Black Cloud*,[28] or streams of energy as in Isaac Asimov's Ames, in his "Eyes Do More Than See".[29] Either way we had better be sure that we ourselves espouse and act according to those values, and try to discover how to be good and attempt to do the best, all things considered. For even if it doesn't quite follow "as the night the day", we may hope that we cannot "then be false to any man"[30] or to any person, even a machine person; and let's hope against hope that they, whoever or whatever they are, think the same.[31]

[28] Fred Hoyle, *The Black Cloud* (Harmondsworth: Penguin, 1971). See also John Harris, *Violence and Responsibility* (London: Routledge & Kegan Paul, 1980), Chapter 1, pp. 4ff.

[29] Isaac Asimov, "Eyes Do More Than See": <http://graphics.stanford.edu/~tolis/toli/other/eyes.html>, accessed 7 December 2014.

[30] William Shakespeare, *Hamlet*, Act 1, Scene 3, lines 79–80. The Arden Shakespeare.

[31] In this chapter I have benefited substantially from useful suggestions from my colleagues Sarah Chan, David Lawrence, and César Palacios-González. I may also have insufficiently acknowledged (although of course I hope not) ideas of theirs that I have come to think of as my own.

Relevant Papers, Chapters, and Reports

John Harris, "As Fire Drives out Fire so Pity, Pity", *Revista Redbioetica/UNESCO*, vol. 1, no. 1 (2010).

John Harris, "Chemical Cognitive Enhancement: Is it Unfair, Unjust, Discriminatory, or Cheating for Healthy Adults to Use Smart Drugs?", in Judy Illes and Barbara J. Sahakian (eds.), *The Oxford Handbook of Neuroethics* (Oxford: Oxford University Press, 2011), pp. 265–72.

John Harris, "'Ethics is for Bad Guys!': Putting the 'Moral' into Moral Enhancement", *Bioethics*, vol. 27, no. 3 (2013): 169–73.

John Harris, "How Narrow the Strait: The God Machine and the Spirit of Liberty", *Cambridge Quarterly of Healthcare Ethics*, vol. 23, no. 3 (2014): 247–60.

John Harris, "Life in the Cloud and Freedom of Speech", *Journal of Medical Ethics*, vol. 39, no. 5 (2013): 307–11.

John Harris, "Moral Enhancement and Freedom", *Bioethics*, vol. 25, no. 2 (2011): 102–11.

John Harris, "Moral Progress and Moral Enhancement", *Bioethics*, vol. 27, no. 5 (2013): 285–90.

John Harris, "Sparrow's Song Revisited", *Journal of Medical Ethics*, vol. 38, no. 1 (2012): 8.

John Harris, "Sparrows, Hedgehogs and Castrati: Reflections on Gender and Enhancement", *Journal of Medical Ethics*, vol. 37, no. 5 (2011): 262–7.

John Harris, "Taking Liberties with Free Fall", *Journal of Medical Ethics*, vol. 40, no. 6 (2014): 371–4.

John Harris, "Taking the 'Human' out of Human Rights", *Cambridge Quarterly of Healthcare Ethics*, vol. 20, no. 1 (2010): 9–20.

John Harris, "The Challenge of Non-Confrontational Ethics", *Cambridge Quarterly of Healthcare Ethics*, vol. 20, no. 2 (2011): 204–16.

John Harris, "The Tragedy of Tragedy", *Revista Redbioetica/UNESCO*, vol. 1, no. 1 (2010).

John Harris, "Time to Exorcise the Cloning Demon", *Cambridge Quarterly of Healthcare Ethics*, vol. 23, no. 1 (2014): 53–62.

John Harris, "What It's Like to be Good", *Cambridge Quarterly of Healthcare Ethics*, vol. 21, no. 3 (2012): 293–305.

Sarah Chan and John Harris, "Adam's Fibroblast? The (Pluri)Potential of iPCs", *Journal of Medical Ethics*, vol. 34, no. 2 (2008): 64–6.

Sarah Chan and John Harris, "Consequentialism without Consequences: Ethics and Embryo Research", *Cambridge Quarterly of Healthcare Ethics*, vol. 19, no. 1 (2010): 61–74

Sarah Chan and John Harris, "Does a Fish Need a Bicycle?" *Cambridge Quarterly of Healthcare Ethics*, vol. 20, no. 3 (2011): 484–92.

Sarah Chan and John Harris, "Free Riders and Pious Sons: Why Science Research Remains Obligatory", *Bioethics*, vol. 23, no. 3 (2009): 161–71.

Sarah Chan and John Harris, "Moral Enhancement and Prosocial Behaviour", *Journal of Medical Ethics*, vol. 37, no. 3 (2011): 130–1.

Annette Dufner and John Harris, "Trust and Altruism: Organ Distribution Scandals—Do They Provide Good Reasons to Refuse Posthumous Donation?" *Journal of Medicine and Philosophy*, in press.

John Harris and Sadie Regmi, "Ageism and Equality", *Journal of Medical Ethics*, vol. 38, no. 5 (2012): 263–6.

César Palacios-González, John Harris, and Giuseppe Testa, "Multiplex Parenting: IVG and the Generations to Come", *Journal of Medical Ethics*, in press.

Catherine Rhodes, John Harris, John Sulston, and Catherine Spanswick, "Provider, Patient and Public Benefits from a NICE Appraisal of Bevacizumab (Avastin)", *Journal of Medical Ethics*, vol. 38, no. 3 (2012): 187–9.

Reports

2008. Co-Author. *Who Owns Science: The Manchester Manifesto*: <http://www.isei.manchester.ac.uk/TheManchesterManifesto.pdf>.

2011. Co-Author. *Animals Containing Human Material.* Report of the Academy of Medical Sciences, July. ISBN 978-1-903401-32-3.

2011. Co-Author. *Neuroscience and the Criminal Law.* Report of The Royal Society, Brainwaves Module 4, RS Policy document 05/11, December. ISBN 978-0-85403-932-6.

2011. Co-Author. *Neuroscience, Society and Policy.* Report of The Royal Society, Brainwaves Module 1, January. ISBN 978-0-85403-879-4. Particularly Chapter 3.3, "Neuroethics", pp. 77–86.

Acknowledgements

This author, like all authors, owes more debts than he can ever hope to repay, some of which he is undoubtedly too ignorant, too unimaginative, or too forgetful to call to mind when repayment is most pressing.

First I would like to thank and pay homage to the wonderful group of scholars who have shared the adventure of creating Manchester University's Institute for Science, Ethics and Innovation with me: John Sulston, Simona Giordano, John Coggon, Amel Alghrani, Catherine Rhodes, Danielle Griffiths, Sadie Regmi, María de Jesús Medina Arellano, Iain Brassington, Alex Mullock, Swati Gola, César Palacios Gonzáles, Gerald Walther, Voo Teck Chuan, Sheelagh McGuinness, Muirean Quigley, Nishat Hyder, Nicola Williams, Paul Muriithi, Antonia Cronin, Anna Pacholczyk, Graeme Holland, Viviana María García Llerena, Annabelle Lever, Daniela Cutas, Sam Walker, Craig Purshouse, Marleen Eijkholt, Becky Bennett, Yonghui Ma, Jasem Tarawneh, and Catherine Spanswick. I wish to thank David Lawrence, who has not only helped run iSEI for the past two years but has made many other contributions to this book which are separately acknowledged in the text. Finally special thanks must go to my colleague Sarah Chan who has not only co-directed iSEI with me virtually from its foundation but is an exemplary academic colleague and leader in every way; full of ideas, a fertile provider of solutions to problems of all sorts, unfailingly positive and constructive, and most importantly, a highly original and creative thinker.

Other Manchester colleagues, past and present, who have been constant and invaluable sources of support and encouragement include Nancy Rothwell, Martin Humphries, and Søren Holm. Margot Brazier in particular has been my colleague, academic mentor, shamefully unpaid legal adviser, and personal friend for most of my bioethical life. Her splendid example has been a constant reminder to me of what it is to be a university teacher and researcher properly so called, an example I have tried, but too often failed, to emulate.

During the time I have been writing this book I have also been directing The Wellcome Trust Strategic Programme in *The Human Body: its scope, limits and future*. Work in that project has certainly fed into his book and I thank the Wellcome Trust for the stimulus and opportunities provided by that programme.

In the same time period I have been a visiting scholar in two other cities and institutions. The first city is Muenster, the second Milano. (What is this "thing" I have with cities beginning with "M"?) In Muenster I was a visiting scholar at the Institut für Ethik, Geschichte und Theorie der Medizin, Universität Münster.

I have benefited in particular from many discussions with Bettina Schöne-Seifert, Annette Dufner, Birgit Beck, Michael Quante, Ludwig Siep, and Barbara Stroop. In Milano I was Visiting Professor of Bioethics at the Dipartimento di Scienze della Salute, University of Milano & Department of Experimental Oncology, European Institute of Oncology (IEO), via Adamello 16-20139 Milano, Italy. There Giuseppe Testa, Giovanni Boniolo, and Silvia Camporesi (who is now at King's College, London) made particularly stimulating colleagues and I continue to benefit from their friendship and advice.

I would like to acknowledge two other long-standing collaborations and one new one. The long-standing collaborations are with the University of Deusto in Bilbao and the Erasmus University of Rotterdam, the more recent collaboration is with ICM (Institut du Cerveau et de la Moelle Épinière) CHU Pitié-Salpêtrière, and Neuroscience Paris Seine Research Centre, Paris. In Bilbao, Carlos María Romeo Casabona and Iñigo de Miguel Beriain at Universidad de Deusto y Universidad del País Vasco/EHU, Bilbao have provided a wonderful environment for doing bioethics and law and have welcomed me on numerous occasions. In Rotterdam, Inez de Beaufort has been an inspiration and a source of wonderful projects and ideas over more years than either of us care to remember. In Paris, Yves Agid, at ICM and member of CCNE (French National Consultative Ethics Committee) and Hervé Chneiweiss of the Neuroscience Paris Seine Research Centre, and at the French National Centre for Scientific Research (CNRS) are embarking with me, Tomi Kushner, and others on a new adventure: "Clinical Neuroethics: Bench to Bedside".

Which brings me to a final acknowledgement to Thomasine (Tomi) Kushner, the Editor of the *Cambridge Quarterly of Healthcare Ethics*. Tomi is a real unsung or more correctly, insufficiently sung, heroine not only of bioethics but of decency and generosity, both of spirit and action. This book is about how to be good, and there is a chapter in it, as you will notice, about mind reading: if Tomi's mind could be properly read and synthesized there would be no need for this book.

Index

Printed and bound by CPI Group (UK) Ltd, Croydon, CR0 4YY